Crossing Borders: Migration, Ethnicity and AIDS

Edited by

Mary Haour-Knipe and Richard Rector

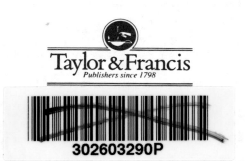

Taylor & Francis
Publishers since 1798

UK	Taylor & Francis Ltd, 1 Gunpowder Square, London EC4A 3DE
USA	Taylor & Francis Inc., 1900 Frost Road, Suite 101, Bristol, PA 19007

First published 1996

A Catalogue Record for this book is available from the British Library

ISBN 0 7484 03779
ISBN 0 7484 03787 pbk

Library of Congress Cataloging-in-Publication Data are available on request

Series cover design by Barking Dog Art
Additional design by Hyberts Design & Type
Typeset in 10/12 pt Baskerville
by Graphicraft Typesetter Ltd, Hong Kong

Printed in Great Britain by SRP Ltd, Exeter

Contents

Contents

Tables and Figures

Foreword I

The societal reaction to epidemics predictably includes strong differentiation between 'us' and 'them'. Throughout history, the arrival of epidemics has been followed closely by an upsurge of popular sentiment directed against whomever the particular society considers the paradigmatic 'other'. These foreigners — whether marginalized by race, religion, national origin — would then bear the brunt of public fear, transformed into anger.

The HIV/AIDS pandemic — its global nature notwithstanding — has provided abundant additional evidence for this seemingly inevitable psycho-social phenomenon. Each country has drawn upon its stock of cultural myths in order to place (or actually, to displace) blame for the epidemic.

Yet, there is a measure of reason to this madness. For with the exception of the relatively small contribution of blood and blood products to the global epidemic, HIV has largely been spread through the movement of people. Nevertheless, while migrants and refugees constitute only a very small part of the human movements through which HIV has become a global epidemic, they are particularly vulnerable to 'other' stigmatization. This results from broader aspects of their societal fragility; often, the rights and dignity of migrants and refugees come last.

From a broader perspective, it has become clear that the HIV/AIDS pandemic, like changes in the global environment, the impact of the global economy, ethnic conflicts, and the problem of overpopulation, points towards a central theme, or challenge of our time. For never before in history has the need to think, communicate and understand across borders — national, ethnic, religious, linguistic, cultural — been so evident. Nothing less than the future of the world is at stake in this quest for recognizing the dignity, integrity and rights of the other, while preserving and strengthening the self.

This book focuses directly on these questions. It is an ambitious book. Thanks to its excellent authorship and creative editorship, it succeeds in bringing forth fresh information and constructive thinking out of the maelstrom of problems around migration and ethnic minorities in a world with AIDS. In this way, this outstanding book makes its contribution to the slow and painful process through which we are all trying to learn how — in the modern world — to be fully human.

Jonathan M. Mann, MD, MPH
François-Xavier Bagnoud Professor of Health and Human Rights
Professor of Epidemiology and International Health
Director, International AIDS Center
Harvard School of Public Health
Boston, Massachusetts, USA

Foreword II

The focus of this book is on the public health response in western societies to the AIDS pandemic, and its implications for social development, including migration and policies concerning migration. It is not a book on migrants as vectors of disease. And rightly so. It would be all too easy to single out migration, or immigrants, as the cause of the problem, and enact barriers to restrict their mobility. This has happened in the past, and has subsequently led to the neglect of other more effective public health measures for limiting the spread and impact of infectious diseases.

The fear that people coming from other countries might bring dangerous contagion into societies is deeply rooted. It has certainly been with us since the Black Death, when in the midst of the fourteenth century a disastrous pandemic could be traced to the arrival of one single ship to a harbour, and when within weeks, the plague could kill up to half of the population.

In the 1980s and 1990s, when western society was still cushioned in the illusion that infectious diseases were under control, the emergence of HIV infection, outbreaks of diphtheria in states of the former Soviet Union, the threat of plague from India, and cases of Ebola fever in Zaire have led to outcries for draconian measures to limit or close down travel, transportation and trade, in the hope of limiting the spread of the contagion.

While such measures undeniably need to be considered in the control of any new or re-emerging infectious disease, the point here is that migrants are not the culprits. Migrants, defined for the sake of simplicity as persons who travel on a one-way ticket, number between one and two million persons per year in the western world. Most of them are regular immigrants to countries which pursue an active immigration policy, such as the US, Canada and Australia. This number represents less than one per cent of the total of international travellers, most of whom are tourists, business people and others on short trips abroad, some pursuing experiences that might well lead to the acquisition of infectious diseases. The annual number of migrants travelling per year corresponds to the number of all other travellers per day.

The focus of this book is on AIDS as a public health challenge in Europe. Its timeliness and importance relate to the challenges posed by providing health services to marginalized groups such as migrants and ethnic minorities. These groups often do not even enter into national population statistics, and when they do, we have ample evidence that they are rarely adequately reached by mainstream services.

This book examines issues of AIDS prevention and care from the point of view of the migrant. Paradoxically, by improving our knowledge and refining our interventions in addressing migrants, ethnic minorities and health, we might at the same time learn to deal more effectively with HIV and AIDS among other marginal groups in society on the one hand, and migrants and their other health and social problems on the other.

Harald Siem, MD
Director of Medical Services of the International Organization for Migration, Chairman of the Executive Committee, International Centre for Migration and Health, Geneva, Switzerland.

Series Editor's Preface

AIDS pays little respect to the sometimes arbitrary geo-political boundaries that separate countries and regions. Within a decade of the identification of HIV, there existed no part of the world untouched or unaffected either by the epidemic itself, or by its wide-reaching social effects. Globally, we now live amongst a myriad of overlapping local epidemics, each with its distinctive character, and each fuelled by different economic, social, cultural and political forces. If such is recognized by increasing numbers of health promotion workers, social researchers and activists, it has as yet to enter the consciousness of many more ordinary people who still seek 'others' to blame for the advent of the epidemic, and for the far-reaching consequences it has had for social and sexual life.

From the earliest days of the epidemic, outsiders and social strangers have been popularly identified as those somehow responsible for AIDS, be they gay men, sex workers, injecting drug users or migrant groups and communities. This book is unique in that it offers a thorough examination of issues affecting migrants, refugees and minority ethnic groups worldwide. Drawing on their wide-ranging professional and personal experience, the editors and authors offer a thorough overview of medical, social and care-related issues. If at times the accounts offered rail against the injustice, hostility and prejudice faced by migrant groups and communities worldwide, they do so because the way we treat others reveals so much about our own humanity in the face of one of the gravest health crises there has been. In *Crossing Borders*, Mary Haour-Knipe and Richard Rector have assembled a hallmark collection of essays that lay the foundations for broader efforts to establish a more socially inclusive response to the epidemic.

Peter Aggleton

Acknowledgments

Many people have gone out of their way to make this book possible, or to make it better than it might otherwise have been. Underlying is the technical and logistical support provided by the University Institute of Social and Preventive Medicine in Lausanne. Our heartfelt thanks go out, in addition, to: Peter Aggleton, Calle Almedal, Michael Arsenault, Ida Balslev-Olesen, Alison Chapman, The Danish AIDS Foundation, Renée Danziger, Françoise Dubois-Arber, Jan Gerstoft, Norbert Gilmore, Robin Gorna, Ruth Gunn-Mota, Georges Haour, Comfort Jegede, Noerine Kaleeba, Merrijoy Kelner, Doris Schopper, Kirsten Madsen, Myriam Maeder, Fred Paccaud, Susan Timberlake, Katarina Tomasevski, Helle Vieen, and to those who have helped us understand, in a way we would not otherwise have done, the different situations of migrants.

But it is to all of the authors that special thanks are due. Edited books are very often preceded by a conference, for which those who make up the book have already gathered their thoughts. In this case there was no conference; all of the papers were developed and written specifically for the volume at the request of the editors. More than half of the authors were working in what for them was a foreign language, and all worked under short deadlines, accepting with grace the editors' demands for extensive revisions at a moment when many had thought the job was finished. None had only their chapters to write: all were fully occupied elsewhere, running programmes, teaching, writing, and assisting migrants with a range of problems related to HIV. Many coped, in addition, with ill health and deaths among those close to them. There were also job changes, computer problems, faults in postal and telephone systems, and in e-mail links.

A personal note in conclusion: AIDS is a field marked with tragedy and with loss. People are still becoming infected. Lives are cut off as people die far too early. No one can be engaged in this field for very long without losing colleagues and friends, and some have lost a great many of the people they had loved.

Yet at the same time there are some good things that have come out of the epidemic. One of them is the unlikely alliances that have been formed, such as that between the editors of this book. Separated by several basic demographic variables, united by the fact that both live as 'foreigners' in Europe as well as by several fundamental ideals; one an academic, for years intellectually fascinated by AIDS, the other an activist, involved in spirit and body mobilizing others around AIDS from the very beginnings of the epidemic: they fell quickly into a mutually supportive friendship. Each learned much from the other, gaining respect for the other's point of view, and in many ways changed in the way they saw the world. One of them has found unexpected reserves of energy and strength to work actively on the book, in spite of failing health and against all predictions, turning negative into creative energy. Out of the tragedy that is AIDS, we want to highlight the friendship that can develop, the solidarity, and the astonishingly powerful resources that can sometimes blossom in the most difficult of times.

Mary Haour-Knipe
Richard Rector

Chapter 1

Introduction

Mary Haour-Knipe and Richard Rector

Migration and HIV/AIDS

Migration and AIDS are two of the crucial social issues facing today's changing world, posing unique difficulties for any discussion of a stigmatized disease, AIDS, and an often stigmatized group, migrants.

Patterns of migration are in a state of considerable flux. Throughout the world, escalating civil unrest, wars, 'ethnic cleansing', ecological changes, economic imbalances, individual search for a better life or just plain restlessness and curiosity, push or pull people to relocate. Migration is a complex phenomenon: people relocate permanently, or temporarily — or they end up staying permanently when they had thought to move temporarily, or vice versa. The ease of modern travel means that many migrants, even if they have permanently left the places in which they were born, will return to visit, perhaps frequently. Migration takes place between continents and countries, and abundant movement also occurs within states. There have been many attempts to regulate migration by legislative means and, sometimes more cordially, numerous studies of the political, economic, and social conditions of migrants.

As for health, we find ourselves at the junction of two currents indeed difficult to reconcile. On one side is commitment to the World Health Organization objective of 'Health for All by the Year 2000', which aims to provide all people with equal opportunity to develop health to the full, and to maintain it. This commitment to social equity implies both equity among nations and equity among the people within each country. On the other side, and particularly in developed countries, we find growing dissatisfaction with the performance of, and escalating cost associated with, health care and social service systems. In many countries such dissatisfaction is leading to talk of rationing of health services and of privatization of some that were once public.

Finally, no reader will need to be reminded of the impact of AIDS. The most complex public health challenge confronting modern society, AIDS has raised basic questions about the rights of individuals versus those of society, about the role of governments, and about the nature of societal responses. The HIV epidemic came at a very inconvenient time indeed, when many countries are having to reduce or freeze their expenditure on health care and on social services. The Global AIDS Policy Coalition has noted that since the beginning of the 1990s there has been a growing gap between the increasing size of the AIDS pandemic and the scale of the response (Mann *et al.* 1992). Most governments are reducing their financial commitment to AIDS, and the political priority afforded the disease is declining.

The extraordinary attention that AIDS has received continues to lack a serious consideration of one of the most vulnerable segments of our societies — the men, women and children residing in what for them is a foreign land. In the published literature, much of the attention devoted to migration and to migrants has been purely epidemiological as, clearly, diseases are carried as people travel across borders (Garrett, 1995). Many of those working in the field of migration, although they feel they should be doing something, may hesitate to use the words 'migration' and 'AIDS' in the same paragraph (Decosas *et al.*, 1995), fearing unfair finger-pointing at those who are all too easy to single out since they are, by definition, not of 'us'. The result is that, in relation to HIV and to AIDS, and until recently, migrants have either been ignored, or they have been overprotected.

It is important to clearly formulate the reasons migration might be of concern in relation to HIV. Migrants are of concern since:

1   They move from one country to another. Migrants are particularly affected by worldwide differences in HIV patterns, and in prevention efforts. Being in a high prevalence country with a low level of HIV awareness can be dangerous.
2   Social inequalities in health persist, and often affect the health of migrants. HIV and AIDS are very much related to such social inequalities in health.
3   The situation of *some* migrants or members of ethnic minorities may lead to potential exposure to risk. Migrants may be exposed to risk because of lack of access to information and to health care, or because of social, economic and legal difficulties that could lead to high risk behaviour (because of legal restrictions on family reunification for instance).
4   Migrants often have linguistic and cultural difficulties in comprehending prevention messages (for example because of different approaches to sexuality) and care-related messages (for example when they misunderstand the meaning of a positive HIV test result). They may also encounter difficulties in relations with key personnel in the host country (health and social service workers for example).

Some migrants may be among the least privileged members of the societies in which they are living, and migrant health often falls between gaps of national health programmes (Bollini and Siem, 1995). As for AIDS, being of minority culture and language, migrants very often miss out on the prevention programmes targeting the general population. In Europe, for example, the first AIDS prevention programmes targeting migrants came into existence around 1990, some five to seven years after those for local general populations (Haour-Knipe, 1991). As for HIV-related care, although migrants are invariably affected as the epidemic expands, and although the experience of other targeting prevention campaigns clearly indicates the importance of uniting prevention and care from the start, programmes taking into account the support needs of migrants affected by HIV/AIDS are still in their infancy (Rector, 1994).

Questions of Definition

But what is meant by the term, 'migrants'? This question arose in 1989 as one of the editors of this book was assessing what was then known about AIDS prevention for migrants in Europe. It came up again as the other was preparing to examine the care needs of migrants affected by HIV and by AIDS. It came up again, repeatedly, as we were editing this book.

One approach to migration and AIDS is to track the effect of population movement on the spread of a virus. This is absolutely *not* the approach of this book. Our aim, instead, is to take the point of view of the migrant, and to examine the issues around AIDS prevention and care in migrant and ethnic minority communities. The definition of just who constitutes a 'migrant' occupied a considerable amount of time and thought, and was an area which was revisited on several occasions in developing this book.

An overruling factor in discussing migration and HIV/AIDS is the migrant's legal status in the host country. This status defines the migrant's basic rights, including those of remaining in the country, and access to health care. Such rights may be different from category to category: for example migrants — workers — may need to have a job and a work permit in order to remain, but others, such as students, may be prohibited from working. In particular, rights to health care vary, not only from category to category, but from country to country. We have reproduced a basic working definition of migrant groups by legal status, and extracted elements of description, from a classification used in a background paper on long-term travel restrictions, produced for the World Health Organization's then Global Programme on AIDS (WHO, 1995).[1]

Mary Haour-Knipe and Richard Rector

Definitions of Legal Categories of Migrants

Legally Admitted Permanent Residents/Immigrants

These are non-nationals entitled to reside indefinitely in a host country. They may or may not be expected to become nationals of the host country, and may have been admitted or permitted to remain as permanent immigrants either because of their individual circumstances, e.g. marriage to a national of the host country, or because of some general policy or agreement, e.g. reciprocal treaty obligations.

Legally Admitted Temporary Migrants

These are non-nationals either seeking entry to, or present in, a country, but who do not have the right to stay indefinitely, and who are not short-term visitors. Temporary migrants often remain in a host country for many years, by seeking regular renewal of their residence and/or work permits. They form a diverse group, including students, visiting scholars, refugees granted temporary asylum, and many migrant workers and accompanying families.

Short-term Visitors

It is difficult to draw a clear distinction between short-term visitors such as tourists, business travellers, conference-goers, and temporary migrants. Short-term visitors are not regarded as residents of the host country, even temporarily, but countries apply varying definitions of visitor status (thirty days or less, sixty days or less etc.).

Illegal Migrants

Illegal migrants include people who have entered the host country legally but remained after expiry of their visa/permit or in breach of its conditions, as well as those who have entered covertly. Some governments tolerate a degree of illegal migration if it suits their purposes, for example by providing cheap labour. In some countries, there are large numbers of long-standing established residents who lack legal status and recognition. Some countries have amnesty programmes under which illegal migrants can apply to become legal immigrants.

Returning Nationals

They include migrant and seasonal workers or students who have completed their work or study abroad, people who have been deported or denied permission to remain in another country, former emigrants who have changed their plans etc.

Refugees

Refugees are a recognized group with special status in international law. The 1951 Convention relating to the Status of Refugees defines a refugee as 'a person who, owing to well founded fear of being persecuted for reasons of race, religion, nationality, membership of a particular social group or political opinion, is outside the country of his/her nationality (or habitual residence, if stateless) and is unable or, owing to such fear, is unwilling to avail himself/herself of its protection'. Recognition as a refugee can be granted by the host country, in accepting an asylum seeker's claim, or by the UN High Commissioner for Refugees.

Asylum-seekers

Asylum-seekers are people who have entered a country or are seeking to enter, and have appealed to the authorities of that country to be recognized as refugees and allowed to remain temporarily or permanently. Their numbers are increasing, especially in Europe. This has led to controversy with concerns on the one hand that genuine applicants are being denied protection from persecution by increasingly tight restrictions, and on the other hand that large numbers of spurious claimants are abusing the system.

Processing applications for asylum can take months or years. During this time the status of the asylum-seeker may be precarious and uncertain — some are detained. In Europe more than 90 per cent of asylum claims are refused. However, the decision occasionally takes so long that by the time a person is refused asylum he or she has developed sufficient ties to the host country to be able to appeal successfully for exceptional permission to stay. People refused asylum may become illegal immigrants, may seek asylum in another country or may return to their home country.

Students

Students are migrants who have been granted permission to stay in a foreign country for the specific purpose of completing a programme or course of study or training. Their permission to remain in the country may be conditional on continuing with this programme or course. Of particular interest are persons coming from developing countries to which they are expected to return on completion of their studies, financed through scholarships awarded by a government or NGO (often in the host country) as a means of promoting development in the country of origin by increasing its supply of skilled or professional workers.

Migrant Workers

The broad definition of the International Convention on the Protection of the Rights of All Migrant Workers and Members of Their Families[2] encompasses not only legal temporary migrants, but also some short-term visitors, permanent immigrants and illegal migrants. The main group of concern is medium- or long-term temporary migrant workers seeking renewal of their residence and/or work permits. Large numbers of such workers are potentially vulnerable to loss of livelihood and settled existence if refused permission to remain in the host country because of HIV infection or AIDS. They are also potentially subject to discrimination after being sent home.

Diplomats

Diplomats are a special group because they are customarily exempted from travel and visa restrictions. Most countries allow similar exemptions for personnel working in the United Nations system.

Necessary as they are, legal classifications do not adequately take into account the second fundamental variable concerning migrants, that of time in the host country. If legal status defines the rights the migrant can expect in the host country, how long they have been there defines, at least in part, to what extent they may be integrated, how well they may master the language spoken, the customs, the tasks and routines of daily living. It is by living in a country for many years that 'migrants' become 'ethnic minorities'. Here, again, both the use of the term 'ethnic minority' (or 'minority ethnic group') and the situation of the people referred to, differs from country to country. Some individuals may be nationals in the country concerned, but easily identifiable because of different skin colour, whilst others remain legally foreigners, but would be impossible to pick out in a crowd. Within the same country, categories often overlap and/or change, as when an asylum seeker is granted refugee status, or when the temporary migrant worker decides (or is granted permission) to stay indefinitely, or to return to the country of origin.

Some further important variables that characterize different migration situations include the reasons behind various waves of migration in a country; the demographic structure of the migrant community (sex, age, marital status and so forth, or place in the life cycle); socio-economic status and education of different migrant groups; and culture. Particularly important for our purposes is the amount of cultural difference existing between guest and host populations: the larger the cultural difference between the two, the greater the possibility of misunderstanding.

These many different situations are referred to throughout the various chapters in this book, which examine in turn asylum seekers, migrant workers, and ethnic minorities. Different authors employ various terms, which we have made no attempt to standardize: thus 'migrant', 'immigrant', 'foreign', 'ethnic minority', and 'minority ethnic' may all refer to the same individual or group in different chapters. What these people share is that they most often live on the margins of the societies in which they dwell, whether they are the multinational corporation executives, diplomats, or military personnel and their families living in suburban subcultures — or whether they are the 'migrants' of which many people more often think, distinguished by culture, socio-economic status and often the colour of their skin. They include, but are most definitely not limited to, some of the world's most vulnerable populations, such as those that have been victim of wars, and those for whom socio-political changes remove all possibilities of maintaining a livelihood by legal means.[3] What perhaps all migrants share is that they, themselves, feel they are somewhat different from those around them, and they are seen by their hosts as being so.

Overview

This, to our knowledge is the first book to have addressed this complex and rapidly changing field. A first decision made when editing and writing it was to maintain, as much as possible, a focus on Europe. There were two main reasons for this. The first was an attempt to avoid a level of generality so broad as to render the book virtually useless. The hope was that if we kept our focus on one region, what we were saying about one specific context could be extrapolated to others. The second reason was to fight against denial, against the tendency to deem that it is the *others* who have the problems of HIV and of AIDS. The publishers of this book have their headquarters in Europe, the editors live and work in Europe. The press and the general public, but also those who run programmes and do research have, consciously or not, been all too ready to talk about AIDS on other continents, to concentrate on the problems elsewhere, sometimes to the detriment of those on their own doorsteps. There has, though, been a certain amount of tension in maintaining the focus on Europe: that we have not been entirely successful reflects perhaps, after all, the extent to which AIDS is a global issue.

The book takes an academic-activist approach, rooted simultaneously in the traditions of research, policy formulation, field work, and activism. The respective styles of these different approaches has been maintained in all of the chapters, which have been edited for language only. Thus some chapters, such as that on legal issues, provide full academic references with extensive notes, whereas others, such as those on care issues and on international networking, are written directly from experience in the field.[4] The chapters discuss the fundamental issues as the authors saw them in the mid-1990s when the book took shape. It documents activities already occurring, and lays the groundwork for the development of AIDS prevention and care programmes for migrants and ethnic minorities for the remainder of the decade.

In the chapter entitled 'Migration Patterns', Charles Westin of Stockholm University in Sweden, sets the stage. If, nowadays, as he notes, practically any part of the globe can be reached by modern transportation within a few days from any given starting point, Westin reminds us that there is nothing new in people migrating: people have been exploring new territories since land bridges formed over much of the Indonesian archipelago. He discusses the roots of today's European migration, including the impact of the Industrial Revolution, the consequences of both world wars, and changes in global economic systems in the 1970s. Westin then sketches macro and micro approaches to why people move, identifying social, environmental, economic, and personal factors behind population movements from country to country. A number of different theoretical perspectives are critically examined. Special attention is given to a review of migration in both eastern and western Europe today, with particular focus on moves to establish what some have called a 'fortress Europe', and the implications of the Schengen agreement.

In the chapter entitled 'Migration, Migration Policy and AIDS', Manuel Carballo and Harald Siem from the International Organisation for Migration in Geneva point out that the rapidity with which migration patterns are changing has caught many countries and regions ill prepared in both immigration policy and in health policy towards immigrants. The authors contrast epidemiological and political rationales for the health screening of immigrants (assessing immigrants' needs in order to be better able to respond, versus screening out people whose health status is thought likely to place burdens on national health care systems). They highlight various risks to migrant health (stress, occupational hazards etc.) and discuss a major contemporary source of preoccupation to policy makers and public health officials alike, tuberculosis. It is in the area of HIV and AIDS, however, that many of the problems and inconsistencies surrounding immigration and health policies have become most evident. The authors remind us of the problems created when people are socially rejected and marginalized, pointing out that some HIV risks for migrants are due to the very policies which seek to control migration, and also of the potential of tourism as a source of HIV transmission. Carballo and Siem conclude that: 'In many ways the coming together of a disease which on the one hand is increasingly reserved for the poor and the socially marginalized, and migrants on the other, is an almost perfect match which symbolizes the challenge before the global community.'

In the chapter 'International Legal and Human Rights Dimensions', Guy Goodwin-Gill of Carlton University, Ottawa, Canada, and the University of Amsterdam, The Netherlands, introduces readers to the premises of international law, explaining sovereignty and equality of states, and distinguishing between national legal systems and international law and obligations. He reminds us that political statements, such as World Health Assembly resolutions and declarations of ministers of health, are non-binding. He then discusses human rights and the principles of non-discrimination, and spells out how these can be applied in the context of AIDS and migration. He discusses the legal and historical basis of immigration controls, setting out the issues for HIV and AIDS quite simply: May states, by way of 'blanket exclusions', deny admission to their territory to those with HIV/AIDS, on the grounds of a threat to the public health of the community or liability for health costs? May states impose a testing requirement for HIV on all who seek entry? Then follows an extensive discussion of current practice in relation to these two questions, using as examples current United States and Canadian policies relating to the testing of would-be immigrants. Goodwin-Gill argues that although states continue to regulate immigration in their own interest, there have been recent movements away from automatic exclusion to a more individualized and nuanced approach, with the issue of human rights coming to the fore. He concludes with recommendations for best practice in relation to HIV screening tests, recommending that no blanket restrictions should be placed on the travel of individuals affected by HIV/AIDS.

In a chapter on 'Migration, Human Factors and Some Moral and Ethical Questions', Lorraine Sherr of the Royal Free Hospital School of Medicine in London, and Calliope Farsides of Keele University in England, explore further the themes of right of movement, restrictions on travel, and testing. They focus particularly on conceptualizations of AIDS as an imported problem, sometimes brought to countries by 'others'. They raise moral questions, especially, around the external sponsorship of research, when studies conducted in countries of high HIV incidence trigger the arrival of treatments that could not otherwise be afforded, and which cannot be maintained once external funding ends. Key questions are asked about the social and economic forces behind migration and HIV-related risk, including a discussion of the notion of 'risk situation' as it applies to migrants, and the specific risks related to the situations of refugees and people seeking asylum. Their chapter briefly discusses current thinking on duties and obligations, and on individuals and communities, as it relates to migration, and concludes with a call for policy makers to go beyond testing and screening to address broader moral questions.

Renée Sabatier of the Southern African AIDS Training Programme in Harare, Zimbabwe, in her chapter 'Migrants and AIDS: Themes of Vulnerability and Resistance' picks up the theme of fear of disease-bringing strangers. She outlines the special vulnerabilities of migrants and minorities to HIV and AIDS, first discussing the social production of AIDS-related stigma, then offering some examples of conditioning factors, deriving from European colonial laws and institutions, which increase migrants' risk of HIV infection. The chapter introduces the theme of migrant resistance resources as an important consideration in the formulation of prevention and care strategies, and argues for the support of programmes which promote social learning on AIDS amongst migrant communities, and which assist the creation and development of peer programmes and community-based organizations.

Oonagh O'Brien of Positively Irish, and Shivananda Khan from the NAZ Project in London, expand on themes of stigma and racism, this time in the European context. The authors compare the way in which racism and prejudice impede work among black (South Asian) and white (Irish) minorities. They describe the specific experience of racism and prejudice, subtle or flagrant, intentional or not, on their respective ethnic groups. They discuss the concern of many members of ethnic minority groups who live in a society which they experience as racist, that to take on board the issues of AIDS would be to ask for trouble; perhaps to invite further prejudice and exclusion from mainstream society. O'Brien and Khan explore the ways in which double layers of marginalization, within British society and within their own communities, affect work in AIDS care and prevention. Charting the way forward, they describe the work of two community-based AIDS service organizations that have emerged from within minority ethnic groups themselves, identifying models of good practice.

In 'HIV/AIDS Prevention Programmes for Migrants and Ethnic Minorities in Europe', Rinske van Duifhuizen of the AIDS and Mobility Project in The Netherlands describes the history HIV/AIDS prevention programmes for migrants and ethnic minorities across western and northern Europe, southern Europe, and central and eastern Europe. She describes the existing experiences, offering practical examples, of individual approaches (ethnic minority telephone hotlines for example), group education approaches, use of ethnic media such as radio programmes, and innovative approaches such as a play for Cape-Verdians which has travelled throughout European countries or a workshop making use of traditional Indian dances and music to develop awareness of HIV. She goes on to discuss the development of appropriate educational material for migrant and ethnic minority communities and the importance of international networking, before sketching out some of the principal outstanding problems. Her chapter concludes with a list of specific recommendations for the establishment of HIV/AIDS programmes for migrants and ethnic minorities.

The ensuing chapter takes up many of the same ideas. 'A National AIDS Prevention Programme for Migrants' by Didier Burgi of the Swiss Federal Public Health Office, and François Fleury of Appartenances in Lausanne, outlines the basis of the Swiss AIDS prevention programme for migrant communities. Oriented towards policy considerations, the chapter offers an overview of questions to which answers must be given in order to be able to implement a prevention programme aimed at migrants and ethnic minorities. It identifies the basic principles, methods and strategies that will permit programme effectiveness and acceptability by both targeted communities *and* relevant authorities in the host country. One such principle, for example, suggests that AIDS prevention programmes towards migrants and ethnic minorities should be part of a global programme, and not conceived of as 'target group work' only. The design of the Swiss programme itself is then described, along with examples of specific interventions. Burgi and Fleury go on to discuss one of the key elements of the programme: the identification and training of health promoters ('cultural mediators') from within migrant communities themselves.

The next two chapters focus on care. In 'Care Issues and Migrants', Maureen Louhenapessy of the Service Social des Etrangers in Brussels describes current work in one of the first programmes to be concerned by AIDS issues among migrant communities. She begins by citing the 'Universal Declaration of the Rights of AIDS and HIV Patients', emphasizing that such rights are all too often infringed when it comes to affected migrants, and also stressing, as have several other authors, the extent to which attitudes and practices felt by the migrant community to be racist can hinder AIDS prevention and support programmes. She then highlights a condition essential to an adequate understanding of the care needs of migrants — the administrative and legal conditions applying to different statuses (not the least of which is access to medical treatment). Louhenapessy then discusses the approaches used towards the programme's clients, many of whom come from vastly different cultures, and a substantial number of whom have benefited from minimal opportunities for formal education. Many examples are discussed: of cultural forms of greeting, of differing interpretations of the origin of illness and of treatment, of AIDS-care needs so basic as to amount to finding adequate food and a place to sleep, of differing approaches to death and to mourning.

In 'Culture in the Clinic', Steffen Jöhncke of HIV-Denmark exposes a central paradox: in a liberal, supportive environment, when responsibility for AIDS is shared by many, it can end up being the responsibility of no one. Jöhncke begins as does the previous author, by defining the context (migrants' legal rights and the structure and availability of services), this time in Denmark, where for both HIV/AIDS and 'foreigners' the policy is towards normalization or integration. He uses interviews with service providers to demonstrate not only miscomprehensions between patient and client, but a tendency to attribute to 'culture' any and all problems with foreign patients. Since 'culture' explains everything, and since one can never know enough about cultures, there is no way forward. Jöhncke closes his article by proposing a very simple solution.

The next part of the book looks at categories of migrant with needs that have to be addressed differently than many others. Alberto Matteelli and Issa El-Hamad of the Spedali Civili in Brescia, Italy, discussing 'Asylum Seekers and Clandestine Populations' concentrate particularly on the latter, reviewing the magnitude of illegal migration in Europe today and what is known about the socio-demographic characteristics and basic health problems of people living without legal rights in European countries. Although, for obvious reasons, we are without epidemiological data concerning HIV and illegal immigrants, Matteelli and El-Hamad review various factors that might render them particularly vulnerable to HIV. Not the least of these risk situations is prostitution and sale of sexual favours. The authors then discuss the work of their clinic in the north of Italy, a rare example where a public health system has taken direct responsibility for the provision of health care services to clandestine populations. They offer a strong argument for the universal provision of basic health services on grounds of public health.

In a chapter examining international prostitution Licia Brussa of the de Graaf Stichting Instituut voor Prostitutie Vraagstukken in Amsterdam, describes the work of TAMPEP, a transnational AIDS/STD prevention project among migrant sex workers in Europe. Working simultaneously in The Netherlands, Italy, Germany and Austria, this is an outreach project addressing the increasing numbers of sex workers from other European countries and other continents. Brussa describes the project's work — through cultural mediators and through peer educators — to develop, implement, and evaluate a wide variety of AIDS prevention programmes and materials. She concludes by touching on the incompatibility between immigration and police policies and practices, and the demands of public health.

In 'International Networking: Building Migrants Networks across Europe' Petra Narimani, Felix Gallé and Jaime Tovar of AKAM in Berlin, address a number of essential issues relating to HIV/AIDS work among migrants. These include the benefits of networking (such as in influencing policy development, sharing information, and overcoming isolation), problems such as the chronic struggle for funds, gaining local support and understanding for international activities and representativity, and network coordination. Narimani, Gallé and Tovar then turn to the field, describing the growing number of European-wide experiences networking and creating migrant's projects, activities which have their origins several years before, but started in earnest around 1992. Their conclusions, tying together the theoretical and the practical halves of their chapter, emphasize the importance of migrant networks for joining efforts, extending ranges of influence, formulating common needs, and consolidating work on human rights and anti-discrimination.

In 'Programme Evaluation' Mary Haour-Knipe of the Institute of Social and Preventive Medicine in Lausanne, Switzerland, and Oonagh O'Brien of Positively Irish in London, discuss the evaluation of AIDS prevention and care programmes for migrants and ethnic minorities. In a new field, they highlight the importance of needs assessment, process evaluation of programmes and services, and well-designed impact evaluations. Using examples from the literature as well as from their own work, the authors discuss various evaluation challenges, such as gaining access to migrant populations, deciphering programme effect and causality, and tensions between programme and evaluation. They conclude with a call for multiple methodologies, for stimulating quality publications, and for indicators of access to services and of solidarity as measures of programme effectiveness.

Notes

1 This classification was taken, with kind permission, from a text prepared as a working set of reference terms for use as background for a consultation on long-term travel restrictions and HIV/AIDS, held at the World Health Organisation in Geneva, 4–6 October 1994.
2 Not yet in force.
3 An European example concerns thousands of young people from developing countries who were recruited as labourers during the 1970s in countries of the former Eastern bloc, and who today are among the first victims of the unemployment that arrived with the fall of the 'Iron curtain' in 1989. As this is being written, the amount of force that should be used in sending several thousands of such people back to their home countries is a subject of painful controversy.
4 Along similar lines, the editors have held lengthy (and fascinating) discussions as to the original sources of some of the quotes used both in our own texts and in some of the manuscripts. World reaction to AIDS has brought forth much fine rhetoric, some of which has been metabolized to the point of leaving behind the person responsible for the formulation of a fine phrase. We have tried to be true to original sources, but must apologize in advance to any who may have originally formulated an idea they find here in somebody else's words.

References

BOLLINI, P. and SIEM, H. (1995) 'No real progress towards equity: Health of migrants and ethnic minorities on the eve of the year 2000', *Social Science and Medicine*, **41**, **6**, pp. 819–28.

Mary Haour-Knipe and Richard Rector

DECOSAS, J., KANE, F., ANARFI, J., SODJI, K. and WAGNER, H. (1995) 'Migration and AIDS', *Lancet,* **346**, pp. 826–8.

GARRETT, L. (1995) *The Coming Plague: Newly Emerging Diseases in a World out of Balance,* London: Penguin Books.

HAOUR-KNIPE, M. (1991) *Assessing AIDS Prevention: Migrants and Travellers Group Final Report.* Lausanne, Switzerland: Institut Universitaire de Médecine Sociale et Préventive, Doc. 72.

MANN, J., TARANTOLA, D. and NETTER, T. (Eds) (1992) *AIDS in the World,* Boston, MA: Harvard University Press.

RECTOR, R. (1994) *Supportive Service Needs of Foreigners Affected by HIV: Acceptable, Available and Equitable,* Copenhagen, Migration, Health and AIDS phase one report to the Commission of the European Communities.

WORLD HEALTH ORGANISATION GLOBAL PROGRAMME ON AIDS (1995) 'Background paper: Long-term travel restrictions and HIV/AIDS', Geneva, 4–6 October 1994.

Chapter 2

Migration Patterns

Charles Westin

It is highly probable that the first humans originated around the lakes of the great Rift valley in eastern Africa. The skeletal remains of humanoids with an upright posture and a brain volume considerably larger than that of the great apes date back one and a half million years *(Homo Erectus)*. For hundreds of thousands of years these humanoids remained in their east African homelands. About 200 000 years ago modern man (*Homo Sapiens*) had developed and populated, though in small numbers, practically all of the Old World.

Historical Perspectives

At the time of the latest great glaciation the ocean level was considerably lower than it is today. Land bridges formed over much of the Indonesian archipelago. Humans crossed the remaining deep water channels in vessels or rafts, finding their way to Australia and settling the continent. Archaeologists now believe that the earliest settlement of Australia took place more than 60 000 years ago. Humans also made their way across the Bering strait into the Americas. Recent archaeological data suggest that human presence in the Americas may date back some 50 000 years. The indigenous American and Australian peoples developed their forms of life, subsistence and culture in isolation of events taking place in the Old World. With the exception of Iceland, the Antarctic and some isolated islands in the southern ocean, virtually all land was inhabited by human groups long before the era of European exploration.

The most recent part of the globe to be settled by humans was Polynesia. This process started as late as some 3 000 years before the present. New Zealand was reached about 1 000 years ago. Easter Island was reached less than a few hundred years before the arrival of the European seafarers. The Polynesians crossed the central Pacific, navigating by the sun and stars, searching for new land to colonize. It stands to reason that these voyages must have been carefully planned. The crossing to Easter Island from central Polynesia, as well as to Hawaii, was a matter of weeks at sea. These sailors must have brought stores with them. The Polynesians represented a modern culture in comparison with the much earlier voyagers to Australia and the Americas. The Polynesians were well acquainted with agriculture and animal husbandry. Their settling of the Pacific islands was a colonizing endeavour and as such a migratory process.

Essentially, human movement over the land masses of the Old and New Worlds in the remote past was a different process. It seems reasonable to conjecture that people who were primarily hunters and gatherers were constantly on the move. Some small portion of all the circular moves that were made by Palaeolithic man in search of food would extend the range of action into hitherto virgin lands. On average, then, the frontier of human presence may have been pushed onward and outward by a magnitude of some kilometres per generation, basically as a side effect of the struggle to find food. Although purposive and instrumental, these nomadic wanderings hardly qualify as migration according to modern understandings.

Shifts of Population

Throughout history extensive movements of population have taken place, during some periods more intensely than during others. Historical records exist of migrations by the Israelites, Phoenicians, Greeks and Romans in colonizing the Mediterranean basin. The Great Migrations that were undertaken by Germanic tribes during the fifth and sixth centuries AD, were triggered by changes in power relations and demographic balances. Slavic peoples followed suit, expanding their territories in eastern Europe. The Celtic cultures on the other hand were pushed back to the Atlantic rim. This redistribution of European peoples eventually led to the collapse of the Roman Empire.

The Islamic expansion, following the death of Mohammed in 632, laid the foundation of the Caliphate. In this vast cultural and political power structure, extending from Spain to the Indus valley, large population shifts took place. The Mongol conquests during the twelfth century had political and demographic repercussions from China to central Europe. Magyars settled the plains of the Danube, and Turks conquered the Byzantine empire.

The European penetration of the Americas gave rise to the largest migration of all times. Slaves from Africa were brought in millions during the eighteenth and early nineteenth centuries. Even larger numbers of

Europeans emigrated voluntarily from a continent ridden by famine, over-population and political oppression, mainly during the nineteenth and early twentieth centuries.

Due to redrawn territorial boundaries in Europe after the Second World War, Germans from areas now ruled by Poland shifted to Germany, and Poles in territories that are now Belarus were resettled in Poland. Another example: 400 000 Karelians resettled in Finland when eastern Karelia was seceded to the USSR. Large population shifts resulted from the decolonization of many developing countries in the 1950s and 1960s, the most dramatic being the partitioning of British India into the states of Pakistan and India (Hindustan) with the subsequent exchange of Muslims and Hindus between Pakistan and India. These examples are some of the many large shifts of population through migration, colonization and war.

There have always been less spectacular flows of people. In pre-industrial society people moved from mountainous and barren regions that could not support growing populations to the fertile plains. Basically these moves were *local*. People also journeyed short distances in search of jobs, trade and new lands to cultivate, on an average seldom more than a few days by foot. Much of all this mobility was *cyclical*, adapted to the yearly round of rural society. Workers would return to their points of departure after harvest. Although international frontiers would be crossed at times, most movements took place within the borders of one state.

The industrial revolution, starting in eighteenth-century England, led to a headlong restructuring of society. Power configurations changed. The rural working classes were uprooted, exploited and victims of widespread poverty. In time, however, as the economic benefits of this fundamental restructuring of society were reaped, gradual improvements of living conditions led to a reduction in infant mortality, in turn giving rise to an immense population increase. Industrialization led to an exodus of labourers from rural villages to growing industrial cities. When child labour eventually was stopped, English industrialists encouraged Irish migrants to enter the workforce. Overseas migration, then, was one side effect of the restructuring of rural into industrial society.

One outcome of the First World War, the Versailles treaty and the revolutionary times following the war, was a prolonged economic decline throughout the 1920s which affected the entire industrialized world. Mass unemployment became a breeding ground for fascist movements, many of which assumed power in Europe. The Second World War, on the other hand, was followed by economic growth that lasted some twenty-five years. All important industrial countries were short of manpower during the 1950s and 1960s, despite the fact that women were joining the labour force in greater numbers than ever before. One important solution was to recruit migrant workers from abroad, predominantly of European origin.

Since the early 1970s countries in the South have been increasingly drawn into the global economic system. Increasing out-migration from these regions to the North is one of the results. Asian migration to Australia, Canada and the United States is intensifying. The main movement into the American economy, however, is from Mexico and the Caribbean. A similar movement is occurring from the Mahgreb and western Asia to Europe. Observers in the developed world are not always aware, however, of the tremendous volume of South to South migration. Accurate assessments of the size of these movements are not available due to faulty or absent border controls. Inter-regional African migration for instance may well be of a magnitude one hundred times larger than out-migration to the North, one reason being that post-colonial state borders rarely coincide with ethnic, linguistic and cultural boundaries. Nowadays, practically every part of the globe can be reached by modern transportation within a few days from any given starting point. One way of looking at it, then, is that migratory movements that take place today qualify as local if we consider the time and effort involved in travelling rather than the distance covered.

Theoretical Perspectives

Migrants are usually fairly young, typically in their twenties or early thirties. They do not represent the poorest or most deprived segments of the population. On the contrary, they are people with resources, initiative and vision. They are aware of cognitive alternatives to the *status quo*. Migrants bring memories, hopes and anticipations. They bring with them experiences of life in a society and culture that differs from the society to which they have come. They usually bring with them a sense of enterprise and an eagerness to work hard and to pay their way. Many may have academic qualifications that are not seen as valid in the receiving country. One thing is certain. Life will change. Although many may realize this intellectually, emotionally they are seldom prepared for the immigration or exile crisis that they inevitably will face.

A central task of migration research is to theorize about why migration takes place. Why do people move, and what are the socio-structural conditions that promote or reduce immigration? Kubat and Hoffmann-Nowotny (1981) have suggested that the key issue is not why people migrate but rather why so many in fact are sedentary. An equally central task of migration research is to deal with the problems of integration, ethnic relations, identity processes and multiculturalism that come with migration.

Theories about migration have been developed within several academic disciplines. Few attempts have been made to synthesize terminologies and frameworks that are employed into coherent statements about the subject matter. One convention is to distinguish between macro (structural, socio-economic) and micro (individual, motivational) perspectives.

Demographic Transition

The most comprehensive macro approach concerns the overall demographic development and its relationship to modernization. In the process of modernization, during which countries progress from low to high stages of economic development, a parallel shift from an initial situation of high birth rates coupled with high death rates to a situation of low birth rates coupled with low death rates will take place. Population growth is low at these two stages because birth and death rates more or less cancel out. During the intermediate transitional stage, death rates decline as a result of improved living conditions and nutrition, inoculations, health care, etc. while birth rates are still comparatively high because behaviour patterns, norms and values with regard to mating, marriage and sexuality take much longer to change. This leads to a phase of rapid population growth that is referred to as 'demographic transition'. Mass migration from Europe to the United States during the nineteenth and early twentieth centuries was sparked by the growing population of Europe during its transitional stages. The existence of an (almost) 'empty' continent to take over was a unique occurrence. Thus, nineteenth-century Europe could export its excess population.

Demographic transition is the outcome of modernization. This involves a complex set of factors relating to the dissemination of knowledge, changing social organization and production, rising demands and economic development mixed with a good deal of ideological justification, ultimately affecting

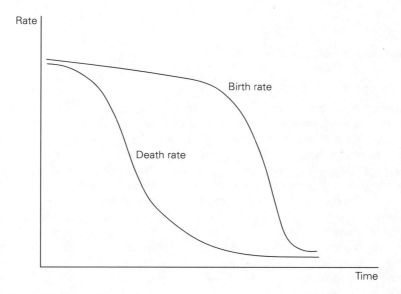

Figure 2.1 *Demographic transition*

general living conditions. Today death rates are decreasing in many developing countries while birth rates are still high, especially in Africa. The world population is increasing rapidly. Almost half of the present developing world population is under fifteen years of age. In 2025 Latin America's population is projected to exceed 750 million. The population of south Asia is estimated to surpass 2.2 billion and that of Africa 1.6 billion. Whereas the global population is projected to increase from some 6 billion today to an estimated 10–11 billion by the middle of the next century when it will even out, the contributions to this growth from Europe, north America, Australia, Japan and China will be insignificant.

The UN population monitoring project forecasts that western Europe and north America will retain their current level of development for the coming thirty years. Low birth rates mean that their populations will barely reproduce themselves. The situation is unlikely to change because the proportion of women in fertile ages is diminishing as populations are ageing. Any increases of the total population will primarily be due to in-migration. The western world will depend upon a trickle of immigration to fill the gaps in workforces. It is unlikely that these will be countries of economic growth. The population of eastern Europe, excluding the Commonwealth of Independent States (CIS), is predicted to increase by 15 million in 2025. The population of the CIS will increase by 75 million for the same period. The main bulk of this increase will be in the central Asian and Caucasian republics. The CIS represents an intermediate stage in the process of demographic transition.

International Migration

Migration is a complex process. It has lifelong effects on the individual migrant with regard to economic situation, political influence, social life, family relations, health and well-being. Emigration affects sending regions in terms of an accumulating impoverishment, loss of qualified professionals, skewed age structures, dwindling investments and a deflating labour market. Immigration also affects receiving regions. There is bound to be increased competition for scarce resources (such as housing), problems of social integration, anomie and alienation, ethnocentrism and xenophobia, as well as an expanding economy. Cultural and linguistic differences between sending and receiving regions will affect the nature of mutual adjustment in significant ways.

A distinction needs to be made between 'spatial mobility' and 'international migration'. There is always a certain amount of spatial mobility within the boundaries of a given state. Moving from a country's peripheral backward regions to its economically and politically dynamic centre resembles international migration in some psychological and social respects; the individual migrant experiences a loss of social networks, lack of recognition, and hardships of establishing himself. Throughout the era of industrialization, rural hinterlands have exported excess manpower to the cities. Nowadays this process of urbanization may involve the crossing of national boundaries, as with the influx of rural Mexicans to metropolitan southern California.

In other essential respects, however, mobility within a given state differs from international migration. A free democratic state does not prevent its citizens from resettling elsewhere within the country. There may be economic hindrances, but that is a different matter. Neither does the state object when citizens wish to emigrate. By way of contrast, legal restrictions exist to the in-migration of non-citizens. Of specific importance are the consequences of state *boundaries, border control, citizenship* and *political rights* when it comes to categorizing individuals and groups with regard to their rights. Henceforth, when I refer to migration I will be concerned with 'international migration'.

The root causes of migration are complex. They involve conditions in the sending as well as receiving countries. Moreover, migration is selective. Therefore analyses of migration need to take individual as well as structural factors into account. At the individual level of analysis, people's motives to migrate, their aims and objectives, their beliefs and access to information, as well as their economic and social means to carry out their intentions are of essential importance. An underlying assumption is that the individual makes rational decisions about migrating and integrating into the receiving society. The individual migrant weighs the pros and cons on the strength of available information (which need not necessarily be correct). Migration may present a means to reach one's goals, be they to marry, reunite the family, seek educational opportunities, find employment, etc. that otherwise would be difficult to attain.

At the structural level, immigration policies, labour market requirements, public opinion, discrimination and segregation, the existence of immigrant communities in the receiving country, and the general structure of opportunities awaiting would-be migrants need to be considered. Macro-structural approaches focus on processes which trigger, direct and sustain migratory flows. Structural analyses generally assume that the economic differentials of the sending and receiving countries determine the overall pattern of migration. If significant income differentials exist between two countries, the flow of migration will be to the country with the higher income levels, all other factors being equal. Factors such as regulation policy, border control and transport facilities confound and disturb the nominally free passage of manpower from one country to another. No matter what personal goals a prospective migrant hopes to achieve, if he is denied entry into the target country there is little he can do but to try elsewhere.

Motivational Approaches

Two central concepts of migration theory are push and pull factors. 'Push factors' apply to conditions in the sending country that induce people to engage in migratory endeavours. Thus, push factors may refer to unemployment, unsatisfactory educational opportunities, unequal career opportunities, discrimination and racism. Push factors include lack of democracy, authoritarian rule, political oppression and violation of human rights. Poverty, overpopulation and environmental disasters are other push factors. Generally speaking, push factors imply that significant numbers are prepared to pay the cost in money, discomfort and effort to seek better opportunities elsewhere. When Idi Amin, the former dictator of Uganda, forced the entire Asian community of Uganda to leave the country, we have a push factor in a blunt literal sense. Likewise 'ethnic cleansing' in the Bosnian war involved the forced expulsion of entire regional populations.

In a sense 'pull factors' are the opposite. If migration is about improving one's lot, receiving countries must be able to offer the migrant such opportunities. Higher wages, lower taxes and career opportunities will always attract a mobile labour force. Social welfare, educational opportunities and public health care in a receiving country are other attracting forces. A majority of the nineteenth-century European migrants to the United States were peasants. The availability of free land to till was a most important pull factor. Nowadays there is no free land to claim. Instead jobs in industry, public services and, in some countries, in the agricultural sector, are the options. In a world of increasing ethnic conflict, civil war and political oppression, democratic government and safe havens will always draw people who are subjected to political persecution, coercion and abuse.

Established immigrant communities in the receiving country represent another pull factor, providing members with various cultural services and attributes to their sense of identity and belongingness. Most importantly, an established immigrant community provides its members with an organizational infrastructure. The community may organize schools, community centres and religious sanctuaries. The newcomer may seek guidance and support, temporary shelter and advice. Agencies may direct newcomers into an unofficial labour market. An immigrant community depends upon an influx of newcomers since there is always a loss of members to mainstream society. Numbers are important if the community is to serve as a pressure group. Numbers are also important for endogamy to be maintained. Since immigration regulations are tight in most target countries today, new members may claim refugee status or apply for family reunification.

Socio-economic Approaches

No generally accepted socio-economic theory of migration has been developed. What we have are theoretical perspectives from various disciplines that are applied to the field of international migration.

Neo-classic Theory

The application of economic theory to the field of international migration has led to various, sometimes conflicting, hypotheses. Neo-classic theory views migration in terms of individual intentions to improve one's lot. Migration is regarded as an investment, the benefits of which will be reaped only much later. The costs of migration should not only be counted in monetary terms but also bearing personal, social and status losses in mind. The frustrations and hardships of the first difficult years should also be taken into account.

The New Economics of Migration

Early neo-classic ideas were expanded by the 'new economics of migration' school. Rural populations in sending countries have rather uncertain and irregular incomes. Sending one or several family members to major cities and even abroad is seen as a strategy for spreading the risks. Migration is one of several means by which households diversify their incomes.

Free Trade Theory

The classic theory of free trade concerns the free movement of capital, goods, persons and ideas. It predicts that economic differentials between countries will level out in the long run. Hence one should expect migration to recede as economic differences between countries even out. One critical comment to this prediction is that the free movement of capital and goods is something very different in actual life to the free movement of people across international boundaries. Countries that are all for free trade may be highly protectionistic as far as in-migration is concerned.

Marxist Theories

Marxist theories view international migration in terms of the global class system, colonialism and neo-imperialism. Instead of levelling out economic differences Marxist theories predict that differentials between impoverished sending countries and exploiting receiving countries will increase and grow acute. Migration is one of many forms of exploitation.

World System Theory

This theory, concerned with structural differences between the developing South and the developed North, claims that the structure of global inequality will remain largely unaffected by international migration. Many economic theories do not recognize the radical changes that permeate the entire society in its transition from an agricultural to an industrial economy. Many policy makers mistakenly assume that international migration originates in poverty, over-population and under-development. World system theory maintains that the development of developing countries is a destabilizing process that *generates emigration* rather than holds it back.

Dual Labour Market

An approach derived from social criticism is the dual, or split labour market theory (also called the cultural division of labour). Ethnically and racially distinct immigrant minorities are directed to a secondary sector of the labour market characterized by lower income levels, insecure jobs and the absence of union organization. A conflict dynamic involving different coalitions of three parties is staged, two against one: expensive labour, cheap labour and capital. When capital encourages the influx of cheap immigrant labour, ethnic antagonism develops between organized (expensive) labour and non-organized (cheap) labour. This is one aspect of racial and ethnic discrimination. On the other hand, when capital and organized (expensive) labour ally themselves, the in-migration of non-domestic cheap labour will be effectively barred by restrictive immigration policies. One outcome in the long run may be the establishment of a caste-type society. Finally, when expensive labour opens its unions to immigrant labour, capital will seek cheap labour elsewhere by moving production to low-wage countries.

Information Networks

Another set of theories relates migration motives to the information dissemination back to the sending country. Migration is a *two-way traffic*. Individuals move in one direction. Images, information, know-how, parcels and money are sent in the other, thus building up a readiness to join friends and relatives who have already left. Entrepreneurs in the immigrant community may actively persuade members of their social networks to migrate. In this way processes of chain migration are established. A considerable share of the emigrants return within the space of a few years, serving as personal conveyors of impressions and ideas. Some commute back and forth for personal as well as business reasons. Receiving and sending countries thus get increasingly entangled into each other through family networks. This approach, though focusing on individual factors, is an intermediary between the micro- and macro-approaches.

Political Approaches

One important shortcoming of the economic approaches is that they seldom incorporate political theory into their models. Immigrants who are permanent residents but not citizens of the receiving country, *denizens* as Hammar (1990) refers to them, represent a democratic deficit. They contribute to the country's economic development but lack political influence. Their interests are not an evident part of the political agenda. Immigration and integration policies, control and security issues, are designed to protect the sovereign state and the interests of its citizens. National interests may thus conflict with universal human rights. One answer is to extend the franchise to those permanent residents who have maintained their native citizenship. Another alternative is to facilitate naturalization and to accept dual citizenship. In most countries of immigration a lot remains to be done in this field. In the long-run, international migration is likely to affect understandings of the sovereign state, its territorial control, boundaries, citizenship and power structures.

Shortcomings

Migration theory may be criticized for its lack of coordination of different explanatory models. Attempts to synthesize various disciplinary approaches are rarely made. For some theoretical statements the empirical foundations seem to be of questionable value. Some economic models do not really apply to the current refugee migration. Many models lack historical depth. Nor do they seriously consider the impact of linguistic, cultural and religious factors.

It has become increasingly difficult to distinguish between economically and politically induced migration. Whereas the democratic welfare states of the North are restrictive about labour migration from the South, these same states have political obligations to grant individual refugees asylum. Instruments of control affect the types and flows of immigrants. Control and regulation policies also bear on public opinion, ethnocentrism and the process of integration. All these dimensions need to be incorporated into the theoretical models.

Gender dimensions of international migration tend to be neglected in traditional theory. Women and children are compelled to accept the migration decided by husbands and fathers. In many cases, labour market opportunities in the receiving country may be favourable to male immigrants but disadvantageous to females. What may be a maximizing of utility to the male head, may be the very opposite to wives and children.

Theories of international migration need to deal with these complex issues in a systematic way. Generative models of economic, political and individual approaches need to be developed and analysed. There is a need for comparative approaches.

Migration in Europe and to Europe

Since the Second World War, the leading industrial countries of western Europe have taken in immigrants. Subjects from former colonies settled in France, The Netherlands and the UK. Belgium, Germany, Sweden and Switzerland were countries of labour immigration in the 1950s and 1960s, recruiting labour primarily from the peripheries of Europe. Southern Europe was then a sending region. Today Italy and Spain are recipient countries for African and Latin American migration.

Many citizens of former British colonies held passports issued by British authorities. They were British subjects and could not be denied entry. As this immigration increased, restrictions were imposed. Belgium, Germany and Switzerland adopted a guest-worker policy. Recruited immigrant labour was not entitled to the basic social rights enjoyed by citizens. In the extreme case guest-workers were even denied the right to bring their families. In Scandinavia, on the other hand, the guest-worker system was never accepted. Immigrant labour tended to be regarded as the embryo of future ethnic minorities in ethnically pluralistic societies.

In Europe manpower immigration came to an end in the early 1970s due to restrictions introduced by all governments. Refugee status and family reunification were thereafter the only valid reasons for granting aliens residential permits. Famines in Africa, wars in the Middle East and political oppression in Latin America led to a growing number of asylum-seekers from Third World countries. Palestinians, Kurds, Iraqis and Iranians were some of the groups seeking entry into countries of western Europe. Until quite recently many states of western Europe have maintained liberal asylum policies. In view of the magnitude of the global refugee problem, and in view of conflicts and oppression prevalent in the world, it is quite reasonable to assume that most asylum-seekers are authentic refugees. Regulation and control policies have had a selecting and directing effect upon the categories of people that migrated.

Putting a stop to manpower immigration in western Europe in the early 1970s may even indirectly have induced developing world refugee immigration. Whereas the economic immigration of the 1950s and 1960s was extremely profitable for the receiving countries, refugee immigration has proven to be much more costly. This is partly due to greater cultural differences and partly because many refugees plan to return once democratic rule is restored in their country, thus blocking their motivation to settle down in the receiving country. For some categories of refugees the wish to return has made many reluctant to naturalize their citizenship, thus forfeiting their political influence in the receiving country.

Refugee immigration to Europe arrived just as the post-war economy of growth had come to an end. Unemployment figures rose steadily and newly arrived immigrants were among those who were hard hit. Although a certain amount of ethnocentrism and xenophobia is probably always present in society, in recent years malignant racism has infested virtually all countries of western Europe. Although still insignificant in numbers, Nazis are consolidating their ranks all over Europe, the main targets of their attacks being immigrants and refugees of non-European origin. Western societies are growing increasingly multicultural as immigrants maintain their ethnic identities, languages and cultural practices, partly because of the barriers they encounter to integrating into mainstream society.

Eastern Europe

Since eastern Europe opened up in 1989, predictions about a mass migration from the East to the West have constantly been made. As yet, however, there is little evidence to support these views. Only a little more than two per thousand people leave the Commonwealth of Independent States (CIS) each year. Before the *perestroika* there was virtually no emigration at all from the USSR. In 1990, nearly half a million diaspora exiles emigrated, the majority of them (60 per cent) were Jews *en route* to Israel. Ethnic Germans 'returning' to Germany (30 per cent) represent another large emigration potential, as do the Pontic Greeks who are making their way to Greece. Internal flows within the CIS are much larger. Russians are returning to Russia from the Asiatic republics. The Red Army is withdrawing from eastern Germany and from the Baltic states.

Minorities displaced during the Stalin-Brezhnev era such as the Crimean Tartars are claiming right to their historical territories. The Roma, a minority of several million in Bulgaria, Rumania, Slovakia and Kosovo, was never recognized by the communist regimes. Massive violence against them in Rumania has produced a mass exodus. Conflicts of the type occurring in the Caucasus and Bosnia may well flare up in Russia or other republics of the CIS. Ethnic conflict and environmental disasters are bound to be a source of potential out-migration from the East.

The affluent countries of western Europe are likely to be target areas for permanent as well as transient immigrants from the South. A significant effect for migration of terminating the Cold War is that new routes into western Europe have opened up from the Middle East and more distant developing countries, through Russia and the Ukraine. In recent years a number of incidents has been reported of asylum-seekers from the Middle East, south Asia and Africa abandoned in small vessels adrift in the Baltic Sea. Excessive income differentials between the western world and countries to the east and south, will attract commercial migrants of a wide range of types, from academics, artists and professionals to opportunists and illegal transients. One aspect of this migration relates to the problem of brain-drain. A completely different aspect relates to criminal activities, a growing traffic in girls for marriage as well as for prostitution, and children for adoption.

Fortress Europe

Due to increasing numbers of asylum seekers, racist actions, economic down-turn and constantly high levels of unemployment, post-industrial western countries are now taking measures to limit the influx of Third World transients. Visas are required. Humanitarian reasons are no longer accepted as grounds for permanent residence. The EU aims to attune national policies on visas, immigration and asylum laws. It aims to coordinate crime prevention and search operations for persons entering Europe illegally.

The implication of a 'safe third country' is that asylum seekers, who pass through a third country *en route* to their destination, will be sent back to this third country if refused entry by the target country. The third country is then responsible for dealing with the situation. Today Poland, the Czech Republic and Hungary are regarded as safe third countries. Thus, migrants primarily heading for Germany, who are intercepted at the Polish-German or Czech-German border, are becoming a growing problem in these countries.

In Bosnia 'ethnic cleansing' has been part of the warfare. Millions of civilians have lost their homes and been displaced. Hundreds of thousands have fled abroad. In the face of this crisis some European states recognize the need for *temporary protection*. Once a sustainable peace has been restored, the objective is to send these refugees back to their country.

'Fortress Europe', or Fortress European Union, is about abolishing borders between the member states of the union, thus encouraging internal labour force migration and limiting or even preventing in-migration from the South and East. This implies efforts to harmonize migration policies within the EU. The Schengen agreement on lifting all border controls between the signatory states requires coordination and integration of migration policies. The outer boundaries facing non-Schengen states will serve as the boundaries of the entire Schengen body. This means that there are no regular or traditional legal means (passport control, customs etc.) to prevent persons who have entered one Schengen state from moving around to other signatory states.

In order to curb illegal immigration, the police authorities will have to engage in more internal control of aliens. This implies that anyone whose right of residence is questioned by the police will be required to produce necessary documentation. It goes without saying that these measures represent an extremely demanding task. Those whose skin colour, facial features and body characteristics depart from the somatic norm images of the majority population are likely to be subjected to increased control. There is reason to believe that these practices may reinforce ethnic and racial discrimination in society. The Schengen agreement is about promoting trade, business and deriving synergetic economic effects from the free movement of capital, goods and people. What is not always spelled out is that shady sides of the economy are also facilitated, such as trafficking in drugs and prostitution, as well as the illegal exploitation of asylum seekers who need to find a safe haven.

Fortress Europe is also about growing opposition to immigration and refugee resettlement. It is about the threatening rise of racism, anti-Semitism and right-wing extremism in Europe today. A key question is whether this turn of public opinion is used as a justification for restrictive immigration policies, or if the restrictive policies in effect are moulding this new opinion.

References

APPLEYARD, R.T. (1991) *International Migration: Challenge for the Nineties*, International Organization for Migration, Geneva.

BLASCHKE, J. (1992) *East–West Migration in Europe and International Aid as a Means to Reduce the Need for Emigration*, Geneva, United Nations High Commissioner for Refugees.

CLELAND, J. and SCOTT, C. (Eds) (1987) *The World Fertility Survey*, Oxford: Oxford University Press.

COHEN, R. (1987) *The New Helots: Migrants in the International Division of Labour*, Aldershot: Gower.

EUROSTAT (1995) *Migration Statistics 1994*, Luxembourg: Office for the Official Publications of the European Communities.

HAMMAR, T. (1990) *Democracy and the Nation State*, Aldershot: Gower.

HAMMAR, T. (1993) 'European migration policies in the light of demographic and migratory trends', paper presented at the Regional Conference Migration Trends, Social Change and Cooperation in the Baltic Region, May 1993, Helsinki, Finland.

HAMMAR, T. and TAMAS, K. (1994) *Migration, Population and Poverty: A Theoretical and Empirical Project on South–North Migration and the Immigration Control Policies of Industrialised Countries*, Stockholm: Centre for Research in International Migration and Ethnic Relations, Stockholm University.

KING, R. (Ed.) (1993) *Mass Migration in Europe: The Legacy and the Future*, London: Belhaven Press.

KRITZ, M.M., KEEFY, C.B. and TOMASI, S.M. (Eds) (1983) *Global Trends in Migration: Theory and Research on International Population Movements*, New York: Center for Migration Studies.

KUBAT, D. and HOFFMANN-NOWOTNY, H.J. (1981) 'Migration: Towards a new paradigm', *International Social Science Journal*, **33**, 2, pp. 307–29.

MARIE, C.-V. (1995) *The EC Member States and Immigration in 1993. Synthesis report 1993: Closed Borders, Stringent Attitudes*, Luxembourg: European Commission.

MASSEY, D.S. (1990) 'The social and economic origins of immigration', *Annals of the American Academy of Political and Social Science*, **510**, pp. 60–72.

MEIJERS, H. *et al.* (1992) Schengen. *Internationalisation of central chapters of the law on aliens, refugees, privacy, security and the police.* Leiden: Stichting NJCM–Boerkerij.

MOCH, L.P. (1992) *Moving Europeans: Migration in Western Europe Since 1650*, Bloomington: Indiana University Press.

SOPEMI (1995) *Trends in International Migration: Annual Report 1994*, Paris: Organisation for Economic Co-operation and Development.

STRAUBHAAR, T. (1988) *On the Economics of International Migration*, Stuttgart: Paul Haupt Verlag.

TILLY, C. (1978) 'Migration in modern European history', in McNEILL, W. and ADAMS, R. (Eds) *Human Migration: Patterns and Policies*, Bloomington: Indiana University Press.

UNITED NATIONS DEPARTMENT OF INTERNATIONAL ECONOMICS AND SOCIAL AFFAIRS, *World Urbanization Prospects 1990* (1991) New York: United Nations.

THE WORLD POPULATION. *Trends and Policies: The 1987 Monitoring Project* (1988) New York: United Nations.

ZOLBERG, A. (1989) 'The next waves: Migration theory for a changing world', *International Migration Review*, **23**, pp. 403–30.

Chapter 3

Migration, Migration Policy and AIDS

Manuel Carballo and Harald Siem

Few communicable diseases have provoked the public fear, political concern, and human wastage as HIV and AIDS. The pandemic has provoked social discrimination and rejection of infected people, and given rise to medical screening procedures which have raised serious human rights and technical concerns. Everywhere, the disease has prompted changes in the way people think about the origin of diseases, their transmission, and what should be done to prevent their spread. Immigration policies and social attitudes to migrants have at times reflected the fears, doubts and confusion surrounding the problem.

Although HIV/AIDS is new, migration is not. An age-old and global socio-demographic process, migration between countries has helped shape most parts of the world. It is likely to continue doing so. What has changed is that rapid communication and transportation systems have made it possible for more people to move further and quicker than ever before. As a result, migration has become an ever more important determinant of social and economic development. Meanwhile, the speed with which sociocultural and ecological distances can be covered has made the role of migration more important than ever in determining individual, community and public health.

But despite the significance of migration, the true size of current global population movement and its impact on both sender and receiving societies remains unclear. While it is estimated that over 100 million people currently live outside their countries of birth, the true figure could be much higher. Official reports placing the annual number of migrants to countries such as the USA, Canada and Australia at one million may also represent a small proportion of the true size of the phenomenon. For if to these official estimates were added all the people who move unofficially, if not clandestinely, the overall total would be much greater. In Europe alone it is estimated that over 100 million border crossings take place each year, and rates of immigration are now beginning to exceed those of traditional receiving countries. As

European border controls become more relaxed, and economic inter-dependence between countries increases, the number of people moving within Europe will also grow, as indeed may the unrecorded illegal movement of people.

The largest and most socially significant migration is nevertheless occurring in developing countries where millions of people continue to move from rural to urban areas. Improved transportation and new travel routes have opened up new market possibilities within and between developing countries. The number of people moving between villages and towns, and across national borders to buy and sell produce has probably never been greater. As new economic alliances develop and as transportation links expand between developing countries, these numbers will probably grow even further.

Internal and international travel has also been boosted by the twentieth-century growth of a multinational tourist industry. Each year millions of people of all ages and backgrounds travel outside their countries for pleasure, exposing themselves and others to new ideas, cultures and ways of life. Tourism has also become increasingly 'off road', taking people into remote ecological areas, bringing into contact people and sociocultural systems that even half a century ago might never have had an opportunity to know of each other's existence.

The twentieth century has also seen a significant increase in uprooting and movement linked to civil and international conflicts. Political persecution has continued to displace hundreds of thousands of individuals, families and communities throughout the world. At the end of 1995, at least 50 million people were thought to be displaced from their homes. Improvements in road, sea and air transport have facilitated their more rapid and wider movement. History suggests that many, if not most, of these displaced people will never return to their homes. Transient and relatively stateless, they continue to live in temporary facilities for long periods of time before eventually moving on again in search of stability and security.

In various ways and with different implications, migration has thus become an increasingly present and dominant part of modern society. Unlikely to decrease in size and spread, it may well become an even more integral part of the regional economy and strategic ties now emerging throughout the world.

Migration and Migration Policies

The significance of migration as a potentially positive force for development, however, has not always been reflected in national policies. Migrants are often seen as more of an economic and cultural threat than a constructive factor, and many immigration policies have remained resistant to them. While most countries have benefited in one way or another from immigration, the political trend in most of them is now more towards controlling and dissuading than encouraging migration. Health status has become one of the means used to define who should or should not be allowed to immigrate, and has served to reinforce the age-old fear that newcomers bring with them new and dangerous diseases. Immigration policies, however, have failed to reflect the fact that many of the diseases which were a cause of concern in the past are now more controllable. Thus, for example, although the incidence and prevalence of tuberculosis is on the increase again, at least in its non-drug-resistant forms it need not be the same public health threat that it used to be.

Important national differences in the rationale for health policies and for screening and testing of immigrants have emerged, however. In some European countries medical screening has become a way of assessing and responding to the health needs of immigrants and has been used more as an epidemiological than as a political tool. Where this has been the case, immigrant health policies have lent themselves more to public health promotion than to the discriminatory selection of immigrants. While it is difficult to generalize, these are many of the same countries which have seen public health as a participatory process determined by better information and a more responsible populace rather than as a static phenomenon to be protected. By extension, immigrants to these countries are likely to be viewed as needing health information and social support in order to help achieve their health and that of the community into which they move.

Elsewhere immigration policies still continue to pose a major obstacle to healthy migration and resettlement. For by imposing exclusion clauses on would-be immigrants (including refugees and asylum seekers), health policies often risk separating families and certainly fostering unnecessary stress on people who have already been compelled to uproot and move because of economic and political reasons.

In general, however, immigration and immigrant health policies reflect prevailing public attitudes and fears. Where immigrants have been perceived as culturally and economically threatening, immigration and related health policies have tended not to recognize the positive role of migration or the special needs of immigrants. Today the idea that immigration could continue to grow at a time when many national economic indicators are stabilizing or receding is forcing ever more stringent entry requirements to be enacted. Growing fears about ethnic imbalances (Simon, 1991; Wihtol-de-Wenden, 1991) and the ever-present tendency for xenophobic public opinion to compete successfully with more technical, political and humanitarian considerations (Wihtol de Wenden, 1991; Lee, 1994; Weidenfeld and Hillenbrand, 1994; Bentley, 1995) is having an impact everywhere. Thus although the real governing factor behind how many people are allowed to immigrate is national economic need (Blaschke and Keles, 1991), absorbability, and taxable benefits to be accrued from a larger labour force (Reubens,

1978), and concerns about the impact immigrants could have on social organization and traditional ways of life are assuming greater prominence in the rationale for immigration policies.

At a global level it is also clear that rapidly changing patterns of international migration have caught some countries ill-prepared. In Europe, which until the second half of the twentieth century was essentially a region of emigration, there are now an estimated 17 million foreign-born people, and the demands for immigration are increasing. Yet because immigration has rarely been considered by most European countries as necessary to their national development, policies and legislation concerning immigration and immigrants have been late in materializing. When they have, they have often been reactive rather than proactive, and repressive/rather than constructive.

Perhaps as a result of reactive immigration philosophies in a region which could clearly benefit from some types of immigration, many of the tensions concerning ethnic-cultural identity on the one hand, and more open mobility (Sussman and Settles, 1993) on the other, are making their presence felt in much the same way as they did in the early immigration policies of traditional receiving countries (Parai, 1975).

The lack of coherence between the reality of immigration and immigration policies is reflected in the differential access immigrants have to social rights, including health care. While in countries such as the United Kingdom and Sweden, specific health policies concerning immigrants' rights have emerged to help ensure equity in health care, other countries such as France and Italy have been slower in developing similar steps and mechanisms (Bollini and Siem, 1995), leaving many immigrants outside the otherwise high coverage provided by the national health schemes of these countries. In Italy, which until recently has been more a country of emigration, the capacity of immigrants to access health and social services has been constrained by economic and legal requirements that were not conceived of with immigrants in mind. And while non-governmental and other charitable organizations have often been able to assume some of the load, immigrants, refugees, and asylum seekers often fail to enjoy the range of services which they need and which they may in fact be paying for in one way or another.

This lack of coherence between emerging immigrant conditions and immigration policies can be highly wasteful of opportunities which come with immigration (Ghirelli, 1991–2; Magni, 1991–2). If only from the point of view of the demographic and economic maintenance of societies, it is widely held that the ageing structure and growing lack of a taxable population base in European countries could be stabilized by an influx of younger people from other regions of the world (Serow, 1982; Arthur and Espenshade, 1988; Ryder, 1993; Weidenfeld and Hillenbrand, 1994). Few immigration policies nevertheless appear to be emerging to recognize and take advantage of this option. Similarly the growing tendency to insist on routine HIV testing of students from developing countries neglects to take into account the fact that many, if not most, of those who may test positive will continue to live productive lives and could contribute to the intellectual and economic development of receiving countries, as well as their own when they return after training.

Legal and economic conditions, however, are only two of the reasons why immigrants often fail to participate equally in the social and health process of the countries to which they move. Other potentially more insidious and pervasive determinants of participation include what may be the migrant's limited capacity to understand what is available and how to have access to it. A combination of linguistic barriers, cultural and social distance from key health-care providers, and the residential segmentation and marginalization that often characterizes early stages of resettlement can seriously reduce the capacity of migrants to enjoy otherwise available facilities and services. In this regard, it is noteworthy that few countries have seen fit to follow Sweden's example of providing special education and counselling to immigrants so that they can participate more actively in their own health and social development as well as in the overall promotion of public health.

Nowhere is this more evident than in the case of clandestine immigrants who, while known to exist and be economically 'useful', are often condemned to officially remain 'non-people' for much of their stay in receiving countries. Coming out of hiding only to work, they are often reluctant to use local services for fear of being found out and deported. As a result they remain marginalized from much of the preventive health work going on in most countries, and rarely benefit from information which could eventually help them avoid health problems, including occupational injuries. Thus at a time when participatory involvement in health is being globally acknowledged as a key to better societal health and to lower costs for tertiary care, barriers to the participation of a sizeable population are being built up.

Although the true extent of the problem is not known, 'pockets' of persistently poor health in countries which otherwise enjoy good levels of health may be reflecting this resultant vulnerability of immigrants, especially illegal ones. In the case of refugees and asylum seekers, the stress associated with being up-rooted, and the family disorganization that often accompanies it, are additionally erosive of their health. Policies and laws concerning asylum seekers and refugees have typically been insensitive to many of these concerns. In some cases, they extend their limbo-like status and stress through laws that state that eligibility to participate in, and benefit from, health-care services cannot be assured until political status is first determined.

Migration and Occupational Health

Among the many health aspects of migration, it is not surprising that occupational safety has become a problem everywhere. In Europe where 'immigration' has often been limited to 'guest-labourers', immigrants have tended to be recruited for jobs that local people will not take. While this has some-times reflected the low status of occupations, it has also been a function of the physical and environmental working conditions characterizing menial occupations. The migration of Italians to Northern European countries in the 1950s and 1960s was initially linked to the demand for coal miners; the early immigration of workers from Pakistan, Bangladesh and India to the United Kingdom was associated with the need for cheap labour in textile industries that were often technically antiquated and unsound from an environmental health perspective. The more recent Turkish immigration to Germany, and to France by North Africans has been equally geared to filling occupations which are avoided by nationals. In this context, clandestine migrants have become increasingly easy prey for employers looking for cheap, unofficial labour which need not meet prescribed safety regulations and other-wise standard employment conditions. The health implications of illegal im-migration can quickly become more serious if they go un-reported and then unattended because of fear of recrimination.

Just as in Australia, where non-English speaking people born outside of the country are at a significantly higher risk of fatal job-related accidents (Corvalan *et al.*, 1994), immigrants to European countries tend to have a higher than 'normal' incidence of work-related accidents. Migrant farm workers are called upon to perform the most strenuous and risk-exposed of tasks and are more likely to be asked to use machinery and pesticides that can be risky to health. Rates of musculoskeletal disorders, kidney and blad-der problems, respiratory and eye diseases, as well as reproductive health problems among migrant farm workers are high. In some regions their chil-dren are also vulnerable; they too become a source of cheap labour, espe-cially in seasonal agricultural industries. In other parts of the world the structured migration of thousands of young women from poor communities and countries has become increasingly associated with almost chronic physi-cal and sexual abuse related problems (Battistella, 1992).

Migration and Psychosocial Health

The culture shock that often accompanies initial contact with a new socio-cultural system can be psychologically complex and involve far more than the simple negation of access to local health and social services. Social integration and then acculturation is a complicated process involving linguis-tic, social, cultural, and conceptual transference processes that can denude migrants of everything they have previously been used to and which may have provided the basis for their identity. The migration of people from rural and often very traditional communities in southern Europe to major industrial cities can equally involve a confrontation of widely different values, expectations, and ways of life. It is a process pregnant with psychological and psychosomatic problems which have remained poorly understood and even less well addressed by receiving countries. They have often been inadequately reported by the migrants themselves for lack of understanding and capacity to express feelings and needs.

Acculturation and the perceived loss of identity by immigrants can also have serious implications for their children. Their capacity to participate fully and actively in the educational process is often adversely affected, as is their mental health. Where associated with the family problems and breakdown that can characterize uprooting and resettlement, it can precipitate behavioural difficulties and crises. In the United States problems of this kind have found their expression in drug abuse among Puerto Rican youth (Velez and Ungemack, 1995), while in Sweden the social isolation of immigrants and problems of acculturation have been linked to higher than average rates of suicide (Ferrada-Noli *et al.*, 1995). In New Zealand it has been associated with frequent and serious debilitating psychological illness, and research findings in Switzerland have suggested a link with difficulties in recovery from otherwise non-problematic injuries and illnesses (Thali *et al.*, 1994). There is also reason to believe that the stress associated with culture conflict can significantly impair immigrants' immune defence systems and place immigrants at even greater vulnerability to disease.

Migration and Tuberculosis

Of the diseases that have preoccupied policy makers and public health officials alike, tuberculosis has been, and still is, among the most important. Worldwide, 2.7 million deaths were linked to tuberculosis in 1992, and WHO predicts another 10 million new infections by the early part of the twenty-first century, saying that over 30 million people could succumb to the disease by the end of the decade. In much of Europe, where over the course of the century socio-economic conditions have combined with the availability of better treatment to produce a consistent decline in the prevalence of tuberculosis, there is now evidence of an increase in the incidence of the disease. No single factor can be held accountable for this re-emergence of tuberculosis as a global threat, but two key characteristics of tuberculosis should be noted. The first is its epidemiological association with poverty, and the fact that it has become more pronounced in developing countries and poor communities. The second is its link to the rural–urban migration which is characterizing developing countries everywhere, and increasingly affecting Europe.

A longitudinal study of tuberculosis notification rates in London (Mangtani *et al.*, 1995) found that immigrants were more likely to be infected than local people, and studies in other parts of the UK have reported similar findings (Sheldon *et al.*, 1993). High rates of tuberculosis have also been reported among migrant workers from South America in Japan (Shigeto *et al.*, 1995), migrant farm workers (*Morbidity and Mortality Weekly Report*, 1992) and Haitians (Malone *et al.*, 1994) in the United States, Asians in Australia (Pang *et al.*, 1994), asylum seekers in Switzerland (Racine-Perreoaud and Zellweger, 1994), migrants to other parts of Europe (Raviglione *et al.*, 1993), Ethiopians in Israel (Greene *et al.*, 1992–3) and immigrant children in Belgium.

The risk of tuberculosis among newcomers, however, is not only linked to the poverty of their backgrounds or to the fact that they often come from tuberculosis endemic areas. It can be as much a function of the environments in which they are compelled to live as immigrants. Their incomes are invariably poor and they often find themselves in overcrowded housing where the spread of disease is greatly enhanced. At times they are also forced to spend long periods in overcrowded and confined quarters while being processed for immigration. A recent report on refugees waiting to be screened in The Netherlands highlighted the role that poor ventilation in the cramped conditions of a so-called 'refugee ship' can play in facilitating the spread of tuberculosis among refugees.

However high (Mangtani *et al.*, 1995) the risk of tuberculosis is among immigrants from poor countries, the European experience nevertheless suggests that the impact on receiving countries need not be adverse. Screening for tuberculosis has proved to yield large numbers of people who can benefit from curative and preventive interventions provided through routine health care. It is therefore all the more important that at-risk individuals be quickly enrolled in what are by now standard and relatively cost effective treatment programmes. In this regard a European Task Force has proposed that international notification systems be set up to assess the overall disease load tuberculosis represents, and that all high risk groups, including immigrants, be screened and provided with access to culturally sensitive care and treatment programmes. The Task Force stressed that because tuberculosis has often been a source of discrimination, screening procedures and legislation should be always seek to enhance voluntary participation in programmes and the self-reporting of symptoms (Van der Stuyft *et al.;* 1993; Asch *et al.*, 1994; Reider *et al.*, 1994).

Migration and Hepatitis B

Hepatitis B continues to be endemic in many parts of the world and is common among immigrants coming from poor backgrounds and regions where water supply and environmental sanitation is poor. These are often the same regions from which people are prompted to move in search of better living conditions and life opportunities. Immigrants from developing countries may thus be at higher risk than migrants from other regions, and certainly at higher risk than people in affluent receiving communities. The risk is especially high in refugee camps where overcrowding and poor environmental conditions are usually difficult to avoid. Because refugees often come from a range of different socio-economic backgrounds, there will usually be a proportion whose vulnerability is greater than others. They all nevertheless tend to be thrust together in temporary situations that often mimic the conditions of poverty and which, in so doing, produce health risks such as Hepatitis B, which are associated with poverty.

Migration and Malaria

As with other diseases, research on malaria has also highlighted the important role played by migration, and has given rise to recommendations concerning the need for screening (Rodriguez-Justiz *et al.*, 1993) and more focused preventive action for migrants (Castilla and Sawzer, 1993). Whether and to what extent the same principles should apply to non-immune tourists who move to, and in, areas of high endemicity before returning home is not clear. But the increasing travel by Europeans to malaria endemic countries, and the growth of 'explorer' tourism away from urban and malaria controlled areas have inevitably exposed many non-immune people, and introduced new risks of return-migration-related spread of malaria. Although the implications for malaria prevention among tourists through appropriate drug prophylaxis and education may appear self-evident, cases of so-called airport malaria suggest how much more still needs to be done.

Just as with tuberculosis and hepatitis, however, it is poverty which stands out as the unifying factor behind population movements and malaria. In developing countries, it is poverty which compels people to accept jobs in ecologically difficult regions, and which drives them to open up malaria-infested forests for purposes of homesteading. And it may well be poverty and poor access to information about malaria control that prevents them from participating actively and consistently in community-based eradication programmes.

Migration and HIV/AIDS

It is in the area of HIV/AIDS, however, that many of the political and social problems surrounding migration have become the most evident. Even though the incidence and prevalence of the problem continues to be skewed by geographic region, new cases of HIV infection and AIDS are now being reported by most countries. HIV is most frequently acquired via sexual contact, and in this sense it may be possible to learn a good deal about its epidemiology from the history of other sexually transmitted diseases. In Europe and the New World, the spread of gonorrhoea and syphilis occurred in the context of rapidly growing human mobility (Shorter, 1992), especially the industrially motivated rural-to-urban migration of the eighteenth and nineteenth centuries. There is no reason to believe that population mobility will not, if indeed it is already not playing a similar role with respect to HIV/AIDS.

The AIDS pandemic has also prompted a more detailed reappraisal of the complex relationship between social and economic conditions on the one hand, and individual and public health on the other. It has highlighted the fact that health and social problems are quickly created when people are socially rejected and marginalized. In so doing, it has also helped focus attention on the implications of marginalizing and forcing people 'underground' because of the way behaviours such as drug abuse and homosexuality are legally defined and socially viewed.

In highlighting this dynamic, the HIV pandemic has also shed new light on the harmful health implications of marginalizing migrants. For the subcultures which drug users and others create are not altogether dissimilar to those which migrants often set up to protect against what they often see as an unsympathetic mainstream society. In the case of HIV/AIDS the tragedy is that social marginalization on the basis of personal behaviour has often coincided and exacerbated the societal marginalization of immigrants, of the poor, and of those whose cultures and sexual preferences are considered 'different'.

In the United States, HIV/AIDS has increasingly become an inner-city phenomenon, primarily affecting poor African-Americans and immigrants from central and south America. It is they who have proved the most vulnerable to a wide variety of health and social problems including poor access to health care and disease prevention programmes. But just as with tuberculosis and other social diseases, the importance of migration for HIV transmission lies not only in the social environmental background of the migrant, but in the social conditions which characterize the process of migration and resettlement itself.

As in earlier historical periods, today's rural-to-urban and South-to-North migration is age and sex selective. Industry favours the young, and developing country labour demands from mining, forestry, agriculture and textiles industries call for either men or women, but rarely both at the same time and in the same location. In the case of international employment, labour needs and immigration policies have often accentuated sexually biased migration by not permitting temporary 'guest-labourers' to move with their families.

Everywhere it is the young, often at the peak of their reproductive and sexual careers, who are most readily displaced through land scarcity, economic deprivation and the call of the city. Their up-rooting and movement to urban centres (Garin *et al.*, 1993) or other countries can involve a dramatic divorce from traditional values and the social control which rural society family structures exercise over sexual behaviour (Carballo *et al.*, 1991; Ecker, 1994). They arrive in urban centres that lack the capacity to economically or socially absorb them, and are often left to innovate or adapt new values that can be inconsistent with the demands of adjustment and resettlement. Emotional vulnerability may lead to temporary solutions in serial and potentially high-risk sexual relationships (Evian, 1993) in which knowledge and use of condoms is deficient (Anarfi, 1993; Carballo and Kenya, 1994). Few programmes have emerged to assist young migrants arriving in cities alone, despite the fact that there is now considerable epidemiological evidence to suggest that the urban poor and young are particularly susceptible to a wide range of communicable diseases including sexually transmitted ones.

Meanwhile, in many countries a typically circular cycle of migration has evolved (Ramasubban, 1992) in which young people move to cities and other places of work, but then make periodic short return visits to their families and communities. When they do so, they renew old social and sexual relationships or establish new ones with local partners. The sexual link they constitute between cities and rural areas may be a significant route of HIV transmission which involves families living in otherwise isolated and low-risk communities (Kane *et al.*, 1993).

Predominantly male emigration from economically poor communities and regions has also contributed to other risks for local women. For where women are left behind to find their own means of survival (and often that of their children), sex work has become an increasingly common option and one of the few sources of employment left open to them (Bassett *et al.*, 1991; Brydon, 1992; Head, 1993). Meanwhile for the men living and working in the predominantly male communities that characterize primary and heavy industries such as mining, construction and forest exploitation, sex workers may be an important vehicle for transmission of HIV and other STDs (Carballo *et al.*, 1991). Most national or regional labour policies have failed to take this dynamic into account and may indirectly be contributing to labour migration-spread HIV.

In parts of Africa, Asia and south America, the spread and spatial distribution of HIV has also been linked to movement along the main transportation routes that are increasingly connecting villages, towns, cities and countries. Road transportation system have become a key component of most national economies, and truck drivers and the sex workers who work along the roads and in truck-service areas have all become potential players in the further transmission of HIV (Ntozi and Lubega, 1992). In Brazil, India, Burkina Faso, Kenya and Tanzania (Broring and Van-Duifhuizen, 1993) prevention projects are beginning to focus on these two occupational groups, but in Europe, where a similar process may be at work, there has been little attention to defining its magnitude and scope, or finding ways of preventing it.

Other types of migration that may have also contributed to the spread of HIV include the movement of military personnel. Heavy troop movements between Tanzania and Uganda in the 1970s are thought to have been a critical factor in the spread of HIV in east and central Africa. Ethnic and political conflicts are thought to have been important factors in spreading HIV/AIDS in Ethiopia (Eshete *et al.*, 1993) and elsewhere on the African continent (Lincoln, 1993; Low *et al.*, 1993). European troop movements may have been equally involved in exposing soldiers, their temporary partners and their families to HIV and other STDs. Prostitution is a common feature of all military situations, but under war conditions the incidence of sexual violence and rape must also be taken into account as a possible source of HIV infection, especially among displaced women.

The latter part of the twentieth century has also seen tourism become a major European industry with millions of people travelling in and out of Europe each year. Relaxed and open to fleeting relationships, tourists are often vulnerable to relatively unplanned and perhaps risky relationships in situations and at times when protection is either difficult or simply not thought of. In addition, however, sex tourism has also become a major and still growing industry. Sex tourists from Europe and other industrialized regions have become an important source of income generation for people in poorer countries and it has become a significant economic asset in many developing countries. As a result, implementing policies to prevent it, or even decelerate its expansion, has been difficult to rationalize with both local populations for whom it is a major earner, or with policy makers who are equally eager to see new sources of income being generated.

Recruiting young people into sex tourism has thus become highly networked and involves both developing and developed countries. Sex workers come and go to established centres of sex tourism from all parts of Asia and Europe. In Thailand where much European sex tourism has been focused, health officials suggest that until a massive prevention campaign was undertaken, up to 1 400 people may be being infected daily. While the estimate may be overly high, the fact remains that sex tourism now involves hundreds of thousands of clients and requires the recruitment and migration of thousands of young women and men from rural areas to vacation centres (Ungphakorn, 1993).

Nevertheless, the risk of STDs in general, and HIV in particular, is not necessarily a function of inadequate information on the part of sex workers. For although many of them come from poor backgrounds, their knowledge about HIV and ways of protecting against it is by now generally high. Contrary to common thinking, it is often the tourists themselves who are either less informed or least prepared/willing to protect themselves and their partners against HIV infection (Hawkes and Hart, 1993). Tourists are thus potential sources of HIV transmission, be it by taking the infection with them to holiday resorts, or by acquiring it there and bringing it back with them.

Nor is return-transmission of HIV limited to clients. Be it with Nepalese girls sold into prostitution in India, young women coming to Thailand from Malaysia, Myanmar and eastern Europe, or women simply moving from one resort to another in search of sex work, there is evidence that once infected and symptomatic, many sex workers choose, or are forced, to return to their communities of origin. Some go because they are expelled from their places of work, while others go back in search of family and social support. Many continue to sell sex or enter into stable relationships with partners who are unaware of their health condition.

Conclusion

Migration of all types involves a range of personal and familial implications, needs, frustrations and difficulties. The fact that people move for economic reasons is often not so much due to 'pull' factors as it is to reasons of 'push'. Pressures on land, unemployment, poor social and living conditions, economic and agricultural crises are but a few of the underlying conditions which contribute to so-called voluntary migration.

In some instances people are able to move with their entire families. In others they move with a small number of relatives, or have to leave alone. The sex and age selectivity of labour migrations, for example, have often shown a capacity to split up families in accordance with industrial-economic pressures and needs. In recent years, many of these needs or constraints have become even more specific. In some cases they have necessitated the migration of female workers who can fit into a growing and predominantly domestic service industry, while in others they have pressured a predominantly male migrant labour force needed to sustain primary industries such as mining, construction and agriculture.

The timing and conditions surrounding population movements also vary. Some people have time to plan and prepare their move, selecting their destinations according to personal interests, plans and a knowledge of the options. Others are confronted with relatively little choice and move under pressure, be it of an economic, political or survival nature. These factors often go on to determine the type of physical move that is made, and certainly help characterize both the perceived and real personal security surrounding migration.

Meanwhile, secular trends have evolved in the dominant patterns of global migration. What were major receiving countries such as the USA,

Canada, and Australia have become less needing of new immigrants and much of the flow has now switched to Europe or has become a South-to-South migration. The attitudes of countries, be they receiving countries or those sending migrants, have also varied over time and have been expressed through various permutations of national policy, legislation, and economic incentive or disincentive programmes. Thus while some countries previously needed and saw fit to promote and facilitate immigration, others have followed more closed-door or highly selective policies. But in almost all countries there have been changes, which for the most part have tended towards the establishment of more restrictive practices.

The reasons that precipitate decisions to uproot and migrate are always complex at each individual and family level. In general a basic typology has emerged over the years in which migration has been broadly distinguished as occurring for so-called economic reasons or for reasons of political persecution and safety. The former has generally been considered to be voluntary migration: the latter has been termed involuntary. Within the former category, illegal and sanctioned migration need to be considered separately; for they present different implications for migrants both during migration and resettlement and social integration. Similarly, in the case of involuntary migration, refugees, internally displaced people and asylum seekers may all be pushed to move under different types of duress and, according to international legal definitions and agreements, their reception and treatment may also vary considerably.

While the typology that has emerged is simplistic, it nevertheless offers an important point of departure in understanding the phenomenon and how the health of migrants is affected. Migration, be it voluntary or involuntary, is rarely easy. It interrupts stability, can break up family life and local social relationships, and almost by definition produces a degree of intergenerational disruption. Migration and the subsequent need to adapt to new sociocultural environments equally requires a process of acculturation which can be difficult and stressful. Old values and ideas need to be shed, and alien ones adopted. Lifestyles have to be changed in order to accommodate new working and interpersonal patterns of life and values. To make it all possible, new languages and repertoires of behaviour have to be quickly learned. The young may be more able to adapt to these pressures than older people and where this is the case, further strains on family life often emerge.

Access to health care and social services may be difficult because either the services are not readily available to migrants, or because they simply do not perceive and understand their availability. All too often the problem is that services are not tailored to accommodate the special characteristics and needs of migrants and in many cases neither the staff nor the structure are seen as user-friendly. In many situations, moreover, social adjustment and integration has to take place in legal environments which are hostile to migrants and which rarely seek to facilitate their successful adjustment. Everywhere there is the tendency to suspect and fear migrants for what they may imply for local social and economic life. They are said to represent threats to jobs, ethnic or social homogeneity and perceived normality and stability.

At the same time, however, the underlying reality is that migration occurs because people feel they cannot function adequately, safely or peacefully where they are. Large-scale migration has traditionally been reserved to the poor and the politically oppressed. Throughout history and all over the world, migrants have often been second-class citizens in their homelands as well as in the countries they have moved to. Be they rural farmers without land, urban dwellers without work, ethnic or political minorities on the wrong side of governing parties, or parents who see the future for their children as unacceptably limited, migrants basically move because they have to.

Meanwhile, civil conflicts, military campaigns and political persecution have become increasingly important factors precipitating migration everywhere. Invariably violent and designed to be socially and culturally destructive, much of contemporary civil conflict has been prompted by the desire to create ethnically 'clean' territories and countries. In their own way they too are the result of a desire to define certain social groups as second class and undesirable. Refugees and displaced persons thus often go into their cycles of uprooting and migration with superimposed definitions of inferiority. Whether they internalize these definitions or not can depend on how they are received elsewhere, but from the perspective of health behaviour and vulnerability to HIV and AIDS, it is important to note that their self-esteem and loci of control are at least temporarily weakened.

Irrespective of the reason for migration, migrants everywhere tend to be initially exploited in their new places of work. Whether it be because there are no jobs available, because the migrant is poorly prepared for better types of work, because regulatory requirements prevent them assuming more senior technical positions, because they have linguistic difficulties, or simply because receiving communities do not wish to allocate them normal opportunities, there is almost always a period of forced 'proletarianization'. While the history of migration to the New World is replete with intergenerational success stories, the real global history of migration has been characterized by tremendous human wastage.

In many ways the confluence of a disease which, on the one hand is increasingly reserved for the poor and the socially marginalized, and migration on the other, symbolizes the challenge before the global community. Progress in defining the risk factors and epidemiology of HIV and AIDS was swift. Its modes of transmission were isolated and defined early in its history. Five years into the pandemic it became evident that HIV infection was eminently preventable. That adequate steps were not taken and may still not have been taken to prevent its further spread is as indicative of the acceptance of a selective human wastage, as it is indicative of the difficulties in changing social environments and human behaviour. Resistance to greater action to prevent and deal with HIV and AIDS has also been coloured by the fact that many of those who have been at greatest risk were already marginalized and hidden, if not indeed forgotten. Just as with many migrants, they too had been set aside.

Human migration and the structured wastage of human resources that comes with it is indicative of the fact that in a world of social and economic inequality, the gap between poor and rich is often implicitly abetted. If there were a true desire to prevent migration, or at least render it less necessary, there would be a much greater and more evident investment in preventing the conditions that make people uproot in the first place. Meanwhile if the migration which has become necessary to some countries from an economic and demographic renewal perspective is to be made healthier and less costly of human lives and social resources, a greater investment will be called in understanding, respecting and meeting the special needs of those who are asked to move. In many ways and for similar reasons, HIV/AIDS and migration are part of a similar continuum which has its source in marginalization from resources, and in discrimination and disrespect for the right of all people to participate as equals in human development.

References

ANARFI, J.K. (1993) 'Sexuality, migration and AIDS in Ghana: A socio-behavioural study', *Health Transition Review*, **3**, Suppl., pp. 45–67.

ARTHUR, W.B. and ESPENSHADE, T.J. (1988) 'Immigration policy and immigrants age', *Population and Development Review*, **14**, 2, pp. 315–26.

ASCH, S., LEAKE, B. and GELBERG, L. (1994) 'Does fear of immigration authorities deter tuberculosis patients from seeking care?', *West-J-Med*, **161**, 4, pp. 373–6.

BASSETT, M.T. and MHLOYI, M. (1991) 'Women and AIDS in Zimbabwe: The making of an epidemic', *International Journal of Health Services*, **21**, 1, pp. 143–56.

BATTISTELLA, G. (1992) 'Migration in 1991: Considerations from a review of the press', *Asian Migrant*, **5**, 1, pp. 4–11.

BENTLEY, S. (1995) 'Merrick and the British campaign to stop immigration: Populist racism and political influence', *Race and Class*, **36**, 3, pp. 57–72.

BLASCHKE, J. and KELES, R. (1991) 'Foreign workers in Germany: Demographic patterns, trends and consequences', *Regional Development Dialogue*, **12**, 3, pp. 127–42.

BOLLINI, P. and SIEM, H. (1995) 'No real progress towards equity: Health of migrants and ethnic minorities on the eve of the year 2000', *Social Science and Medicine*, **41**, 6, pp. 819–28.

BRORING, G. and VAN-DUIFHUIZEN, R. (1993) 'Mobility and the spread of HIV/AIDS: A challenge to health promotion' (editorial), *AIDS Health Promotion Exchange*, **1**, pp. 1–3.

BRYDON, L. (1992) 'Ghanaian women in the migration process', in GHANT, S. (Ed.) *Gender and Migration in Developing Countries*, pp. 91–108, London: Belhaven Press.

CARBALLO, M. and KENYA, P.I. (1994) 'Behavioral issues and AIDS', in ESSEX M. *et al.* (Eds) *AIDS in Africa*, pp. 497–513, New York: Raven Press.

CARBALLO, M., TAWIL, O. and HOLMES, K. (1991) 'Sexual behaviour: Temporal and cross-cultural trends', in WASSERHEITH, J.N. *et al.* (Eds) *Research Issues in Human Behaviour and Sexually Transmitted Diseases in the AIDS Area*, pp. 122–40, Washington: American Society for Microbiology.

CASTILLA, R.E. and SAWZER, D.O. (1993) 'Malaria rates and fate: A socio-democratic study of malaria in Brazil', *Social Science and Medicine*, **37**, 9, pp. 1137–45.

CORVALAN, C.F., DRISCOLL, T.R. and HARRISON, J.E. (1994) 'Role of migrant factors in work-related fatalities in Australia', *Scandinavian Journal of Work and Environmental Health*, **20**, 5, pp. 364–70.

DECLUDT, B., PECOUL, B., BIBERSON, P., LANG, R. and IMIVITHAYA, S. (1991) *Malaria surveillance among the displaced Karen population in Thailand, April 1984 to February 1989, Mae Sot, Thailand*, **22**, 4, pp. 504–8.

ECKER, N. (1994) 'Culture and sexual scripts out of Africa: A North American trainer's view of taboos, tradition, trouble and truth', *Siecus Report*, **22**, 2, pp. 16–21.

ESHETE, H., HEAST, N., LINDAN, K. and MANDEL, J. (1993) 'Ethnic conflicts, poverty and AIDS in Ethiopia', (letter) *Lancet*, 8 May, **341**, 8854, p. 1219.

EVIAN, C. (1993) 'AIDS and the cycle of poverty', *Nursing RSA*, **8**, 1, p. 45.

FERRADA-NOLI, M., ASBERG, M., ORMSTAD, K. and NORDSTROM, P. (1995) 'Definite and undetermined forensic diagnoses of suicide among immigrants in Sweden', *Acta Psychiatrica Scandinavica*, **91**, 2, pp. 130–5.

GARIN, B., JEANNEL, D., KAZADI, K., COMBE, P., SINGA, L. and DE-THE, G. (1993) 'Introduction of HIV-1 in a rural city of Zaire', *Annales de la Société Belge de Médecine Tropicale*, **73**, 2, pp. 143–7.

GHIRELLI, M. (1991–2) 'Europe without; L'Europa senza', *Critica Sociologica*, **100–1**, pp. 90–6.

GREENE, V.W., DOLBERG, O.T., ALKAN, M.L. and SCHLAEFFER, F.C. (1992–3) 'Tuberculosis cases in the Negev 1978–1987: Ethnicity, sex and age', *Public Health Review*, **20**, 1–2, pp. 53–60.

HAWKES, S.J. and HART, G.J. (1993) 'Travel, migration and HIV', *AIDS Care*, **5**, 2, pp. 207–14.

HEAD, J. (1993) 'Behavioural assumptions about the spread of HIV: A reply to Helen Schneider', *AIDS Bulletin*, **2**, 2, pp. 18–19.

'HIV infection, syphilis and tuberculosis screening among migrant farm workers in Florida' (1992), *Morbidity and Mortality Weekly Report*, **41**, 39, pp. 723–5.

KANE, F., ALARY, M., NDOYE, I., COLL, A.M., M'BOUB, S., GUEYE, A., KANKI, P.J. and JOLY, J.R. (1993) 'Temporary expatriation is related to HIV-1 infection in rural Senegal', *AIDS*, **7**, 9, pp. 1261–5.

KIDSON, C. (1993) 'Trade, population flow and transnation malaria control', *Southeast Asia Journal of Tropical Medicine and Public Health*, **24**, 2, pp. 213–15.

LEE, D. (1994) 'No refugees please, We're British', *New Statesman and Society*, **7**, 311, pp. 22–3.

LINCOLN, D.W. (1993) 'Reproductive health, population growth, economic development and environmental change', *CIBA Foundation Symposium*, **175**, pp. 197–214.

LOW, N., EGGER, M., GORTER, A., SANDIFORD, P., GONZALEZ, A., PAUW, J., FERRIE, J. and DAVEY-SMITH, G. (1993) 'AIDS in Nicaragua: Epidemiological, political and sociocultural perspectives', *International Journal of Health Services*, **23**, 4, pp. 685–702.

MAGNI, R. (1991–2) 'Europe: Better goods than people?' (Europa: meglio merci che persone?), *Critica Sociologica*, **100–1**, pp. 97–102.

MALONE, J.L., PAPARELLO, S.F., MALONE, J.D., HILL, H.E., CONRAD, K.A., MYERS, J.W., LILLIBRIDGE, S.R. and WEILL, P.J. (1994) 'Drug susceptibility of mycobacterium tuberculosis isolates from recent Haitian migrants: Correlation with clinical response', *Clin-Infect-Disease*, **19**, 5, pp. 938–40.

MANGTANI, P., JOLLEY, D.J., WATSON, J.M. and RODRIGUES, L.C. (1995) 'Socio-economic deprivation and notification rates for tuberculosis in London during 1982–91', *British Medical Journal*, **310**, 6985, pp. 963–6.

NTOZI, J. and LUBEGA, M. (1992) 'Patterns of sexual behaviour and the spread of AIDS in Uganda', in DYSON, T. (Ed.) *Sexual Behaviour and Networking: Anthropological and Socio-cultural Studies on the Transmission of HIV*, pp. 315–33, Liège: Derouaux-Ordina.

PANG, S.C., HARRISON, R.H., CLAYTON, A.S., MERCER, J. and BREARLEY, J. (1994) 'Tuberculosis case-finding in Western Australia', *Resp-Med*, **88**, 3, pp. 213–17.

PARAI, L. (1975) 'Canada's immigration policy, 1962–74', *International Migration Review*, **9**, 4, 32, pp. 449–77.

RACINE-PERREOAUD, E. and ZELLWEGER, J.P. (1994) 'Preventive antituberculosis chemotherapy in 250 patients of the antituberculosis outpatient clinic in Lausanne', *Schweiz-Med-Wochenschr*, **124**, 17, pp. 705–11.

RAMASUBBAN, R. (1992) 'Sexual behaviour and conditions of health care: Potential risks for HIV transmission in India', in DYSON, T. (Ed.) *Sexual Behaviour and Networking: Anthropological and Socio-cultural Studies on the Transmission of HIV*, pp. 175–202, Liège: Derouaux-Ordina.

RAVIGLIONE, M.C., SUDRE, P., RIEDER, H.L., SPINACI, S. and KOCHI, A. (1993) 'Secular trends of tuberculosis in Western Europe', *Bulletin of the World Health Organization*, **71**, 3–4, pp. 297–306.

REIDER, H.L., ZELLWEGER, J.P., RAVIGLIONE, M.C., KEIZER, S.T. and MIGLIORI, G.B. (1994) 'Tuberculosis control in Europe and international migration', *Eur-Resp-J*, **7**, 8, pp. 1545–53.

REUBENS, E.P. (1978) 'Aliens, jobs and immigration policy', *Public Interest*, **51**, pp. 113–34.

RODRIGUEZ-JUSTIZ, F., FERNANDEZ-NUNEZ, A., MARTINEZ-SANCHEZ, R. and DIAZ-JIDY, M. (1993) 'International health monitoring: Special screening among foreign grant recipients at their arrival in Cuba', *Rev-Cub-Med-Trop*, **45**, 1, pp. 52–62.

RYDER, N.B. (1993) 'Reflections on replacement', *Family Planning Perspectives*, **25**, 6, pp. 273–7.

SEROW, W.J. (1982) 'The effects of an aging population on immigration policy', *Journal of Applied Gerontology*, **1**, pp. 26–33.

SHELDON, C.D., PROBERT, C.S., COCK, H., KING, K., RAMPTON, D.S., BARNES, N.C. and MAYBURRY, J.F. (1993) 'Incidence of abdominal tuberculosis in Bangladeshi migrants in East London', *Tuber-Lung Disease*, **74**, 1, pp. 12–15.

SHIGETO, E., SATO, H., SHIGETO, N., KAMADA, T., ABE, C., TAKAHASHI, M. and MORI,

T. (1995) 'An outbreak of tuberculosis involving foreign workers from South America', *Kekkaku*, May, **70**, 5, pp. 347–54.

SHORTER, E. (1992) 'What can two historical examples of sexually transmitted diseases teach us about AIDS', in TYSON, T. (Ed.) *Social Behaviour and Networking: Anthropological and Socio-cultural Studies on the Transmission of HIV*, pp. 49–64, Liège: Derouaux-Ordina.

SIMON, G. (1991) 'France: A land of long-time yet unrecognized immigration', *Regional Development-Dialogue*, **12**, 3, pp. 115–26.

SUSSMAN, M. and SETTLES, B.H. (1993) 'Policy and research issues regarding family mobility and immigration', *Marriage and Family Review*, **19**, 3–4, pp. 209–32.

THALI, A., STERN, S., ROTHENBUHLER, B. and KRAAN, K. (1994) 'The role of psychosocial factors in a chronic course after injuries of the lower spine', *Z-Unfallchir-Versicherungsmed.*, April, **87**, 1, pp. 31–44.

UNGPHAKORN, J. (1993) 'The impact of AIDS on women in Thailand', in BERER, M. and RAY, S. (Eds) *Women and HIV/AIDS: An International Resource Book. Information, Action and Resources on Women and HIV/AIDS, Reproductive Health and Sexual Relationships*, pp. 56–7, London: Pandora Press.

VAN DER STUYFT, P., WOODWARD, M., AMSTRONG, J. and DE MUYNCK, A. (1993) 'Uptake of preventive health care among Mediterranean migrants in Belgium', *Journal of Epidemiology and Community Health*, **47**, 1, pp. 3–10.

VELEZ, C.N. and UNGEMACK, J.A. (1995) 'Psychosocial correlates of drug use among Puerto Rican Youth: Generational status differences', *Social Science and Medicine*, **40**, 1, pp. 91–103.

WEIDENFELD, W. and HILLENBRAND, O. (1994) 'EC immigration policy: Challenges, options, consequences' (EG Einwanderungspolitik: Herausforderungen, Optionen, Folgen), *Internationale Politik und Gesellschaft*, **1**, pp. 31–9.

WIHTOL-DE-WENDEN, C. (1991) 'Immigration policy and the issue of nationality', *Ethnic and Racial Studies*, **14**, 3, pp. 319–32.

Chapter 4

AIDS and HIV, Migrants and Refugees:
International Legal and Human Rights Dimensions

Guy S. Goodwin-Gill[1]

The modern notion of the nation-state invariably begins and often ends with the reference point of 'membership', for communities commonly define themselves by contrast with, or in opposition to, others. The shades of difference, actual or perceived, emerge in denial of the right to emigrate or of entitlement to enter elsewhere, notwithstanding article 13(2) of the 1948 Universal Declaration of Human Rights and article 12(2) of the 1966 Covenant on Civil and Political Rights, both of which proclaim the freedom of movement. The fact of control over the movement of persons, and particularly over the entry and residence of non-citizens, invites attention to the role of international law in this area of state authority, and in other domains in which differential treatment is accorded to anyone, whether citizen or not.

Early immigration controls were developed to exclude criminals, but were soon extended to the potential 'social charge', the sick and the disabled, and the politically undesirable. Countries receiving substantial immigration at that time also incorporated racial bases for exclusion, intended to maintain the dominant north European characteristics of their societies (Plender, 1988, pp. 66–75). Those few countries, such as Canada, that are still 'immigration countries' today, recognize that immigration can meet the needs and aspirations of resident communities by facilitating the strengthening of family and cultural links; and that it satisfies domestic concerns and international obligations with respect to refugees.

For the most part, however, immigration policy today is characterized by controls that serve narrowly defined national goals. Western European countries officially turned off the immigration flow in the early 1970s, at a time of economic recession, and it has never been officially restarted, even though many European states are effectively multicultural societies with substantial domestic ties overseas (Hammar, 1985; Castles *et al.*, 1984). Up till now, international law has played a small role in this contentious area, but the HIV/AIDS pandemic and states' responses invite closer attention to the prevalence and impact of international standards.

International Law

International law primarily governs the legal relations between states, discrete units each otherwise responsible to themselves for economic, social, cultural or political matters. Only relatively recently has international law begun to provide a basis for the protection of the rights of individuals. One unique aspect of the international legal regime, which distinguishes it from national legal systems, is the phenomenon of state sovereignty. International law, in principle, is founded on the doctrine of the equality and independence of states. There is *no* central legislature, *no* automatic compulsory jurisdiction, and in regard to many 'internal' matters, states may claim a free hand and will be presumed (by other states) to enjoy exclusive authority.

Sovereignty and the equality of states represent the basic constitutional doctrine of the law of nations (UN Charter, arts. 2[1], 2[4] and 2[7]), generally comprising, *prima facie* exclusive jurisdiction over a territory and the permanent population living there; the duty of non-intervention in the area of exclusive jurisdiction of other states; and the dependence of obligations arising from customary international law and from treaty upon the consent of the state. Consent remains important, but a state is not free to unilaterally withdraw its consent to an obligation otherwise accepted. Its participation in the international system is premised on acceptance of certain essentially non-negotiable ground rules. Within the bounds set by international law, sovereignty implies, among other matters, the capacity to regulate the entry and activities of non-nationals, and generally to be the bearer of international rights and duties.

International law also differs from national legal systems in its primary sources. Treaties and custom are the most common primary sources. 'Treaties' are agreements voluntarily and formally undertaken with another state or states, usually on a basis of reciprocity. Like contractual relationships in domestic law, they may create rights and obligations, or set standards, and they may be called covenants, conventions, or protocols. In principle, treaties 'bind' only the 'parties', that is, those states which have *signed* and *ratified* the text. The rules they reflect or consolidate, however, may come to bind non-parties, for example as customary international law. 'Custom' in this context refers to the fact of a practice followed by states in the persuasion that it is binding; here, what states actually do is what counts, and when what they do ceases to be mere usage, but becomes a practice followed under the conviction that it must be, so we have a rule of customary international law.

International obligations, like international law itself, may be bilateral (between two states), multilateral (between three or more states, either at the universal or regional level), or complex (for example, where they are linked to the creation of international institutions, such as the United Nations, the World Health Organization, or the European Union); they also may have their source in treaty or custom. International law and obligations are to be distinguished from non-binding political statements, declarations and resolutions. Advocates are often tempted to base arguments on resolutions of the UN General Assembly or other similar bodies, particularly when these have been adopted unanimously or by consensus. General Assembly resolutions, however, do *not* create binding obligations for states; they are recommendations at best, but may point the way to emerging standards.

International Law and National Law

Does one legal system prevail over the other? Can international law invalidate municipal law? Common sense says no; invalidity and liability are separable. A well-settled rule of international law lays down that a state cannot plead the inadequacy of its own law in justification of its failure to meet international standards. Merely failing to bring national law into line with international standards is not usually a breach in itself, which only arises when there is a violation in a specific instance.

Treaties can (generally) only be 'enforced' by national courts if they have been incorporated into domestic law, at least in countries following the common law tradition. The distinction between 'enforcement' in national law and compliance with international obligations must be clearly understood. Whether a treaty is incorporated is a relevant factor, but whether municipal law and practice satisfy international legal obligations is another matter entirely, and a question of fact to be determined by international law. A long line of authority confirms the principle that, when state responsibility is at issue, international law prevails over national law.

Human Rights

Over the last fifty years, international law has increasingly recognized 'human rights' as a body of rules, principles and standards, generally benefitting individuals, which states are obliged to respect and protect. Basic human rights derive their force from customary international law, and indicate the content of the *general* obligations which control and structure the treatment by states of nationals and aliens. Human rights treaties indicate more precisely the types of obligations that states have accepted with regard to such treatment. Particularly important are those instruments of universal or potentially universal application which incorporate a supervisory or treaty-monitoring mechanism, such as the 1966 Covenants on Civil and Political Rights, and on Economic, Social and Cultural Rights; the 1984 Convention against Torture; and the 1989 Convention on the Rights of the Child (Alston, 1992).

Article 2(1) of the Covenant on Civil and Political Rights is a representative provision obliging the state to respect and to ensure the rights declared to 'all individuals within its territory and subject to its jurisdiction'. The same article elaborates a principle of non-discrimination in broad terms, including national or social origin, birth or other status, within the list of prohibited grounds of distinction. While states may derogate from some obligations in certain exceptional circumstances, such as a public emergency threatening the life of the nation, any such measures must be consistent with states' other obligations under international law, and no derogation is allowed from those provisions which guarantee the right to life, or which forbid torture or inhuman treatment, slavery, servitude, or conviction or punishment under retroactive laws, or which guarantee the right to recognition as a person before the law and the right to freedom of conscience, thought and religion. The Covenant has been widely ratified, and many rights also enjoy a positive foundation in general international law.

Refugees are entitled to special protection (Goodwin-Gill, 1996). The most important international legal instruments are the 1951 Convention and the 1967 Protocol relating to the Status of Refugees, to which 131 states have acceded, and states are bound in particular by the principle of *non-refoulement* which requires that they not return a refugee to a country in which he or she may face persecution. This rule is generally understood also to include the principle of non-rejection at the frontier, and to extend equally to 'asylum seekers', pending a decision on their claim to be in need of international protection. Although there is no legal obligation to grant asylum to refugees, in the sense of a permanent solution, many countries do grant admission or residence to those recognized as having a well-founded fear of persecution or at risk of other relevant violation of their human rights.

The Principle of Non-discrimination

The 1948 Universal Declaration of Human Rights opens in Article 1 with the affirmative, 'All human beings are born free and equal in dignity and rights'. The Preamble to the United Nations Charter proclaims the determination 'to reaffirm faith in fundamental human rights, in the dignity and worth of the human person'; and as one human rights advocate observed, 'it is the recognition that all human beings differ from each other, and that each individual is unique, which underlies the concept of the integrity and dignity of the individual person which human rights law is primarily concerned to protect' (Sieghart, 1983, s.1.10).

In human rights law and practice, the principle of non-discrimination is a constant and fundamental premise. This chapter seeks to analyse those provisions which appear to permit differential treatment, particularly on the basis of health status. It focuses on the rationale and justification for such distinctions, and assesses to what extent they may be valid or invalid according to international standards. The principle of non-discrimination places on those who would make distinctions in the recognition or protection of rights, the burden of showing that any particular status is a relevant basis for differentiation; that the distinction is implemented in pursuit of a reasonable aim or objective; that it is necessary, no alternative action being available; and that the discriminatory measures taken or contemplated are proportional to the end to be achieved.

International law recognizes the continuing authority of the state to distinguish between citizens and non-citizens in certain areas. Fundamental rights, however, permit no such distinctions, while others require a measure of protection that both excludes arbitrary discrimination and best preserves human dignity and integrity. Unreasoning and unreasonable distinctions are prohibited in general human rights instruments, and in others dealing with specific freedoms. Even where exceptions may be made, international law standards regulate the exercise of state powers. Thus, while economic self-interest offers one basis for control over entry (not necessarily controversial, but not absolute either), alone it hardly justifies the refusal of family reunification.

The Movements of People between States

Migrants and refugees have a strong interest in liberty and personal integrity rights, including freedom of movement, the right to leave and to return to one's own country, to enter another country, not to be expelled, and not to be returned to a country in which life or freedom may be endangered. Procedural guarantees, which offer the basis and opportunity to claim or defend rights, are also important, and include equal protection of the law, as well as access to courts and remedies. In the migration context, status rights play a significant role, for example, the rights that accrue to the resident or the refugee with asylum; the right of the child to a nationality; the rights of the family to reunification and of children to special protection.

A coherent analysis must take into account the factual situation within which rules operate, change and develop, as well as the entitlements and interests of national or host communities, bearing in mind the frequently conditional or qualified nature of many human rights. Membership in a given community is fundamental, but competing equities can never be entirely discounted, such as those that arise from long residence, from the facts of relationship, or from situations of distress or humanitarian necessity. In practice, however, migrants, refugees and asylum seekers often remain on the periphery of effective protection. Non-nationals, simply because of their lack of citizenship, are perceived to stand outside the community, and on that basis may be denied the substantive and procedural entitlements normally accorded to members.

Immigration Controls

The increase in scientific knowledge and an enhanced capacity to treat disease have seen automatic barriers to the admission of non-nationals gradually replaced by a more refined approach. The European Community, for example, is premised on, among others, the principles of free movement of labour and freedom of establishment, which in turn presuppose a moderation or elimination of the controls normally exercised by Member States with respect to the nationals of other Member States, including restrictions on entry. Council Directive 64/221/EEC seeks to promote coordination in the areas of public policy, public security and public health, by listing the *only* diseases or disabilities that may justify refusal of entry, and also by providing for legal remedies on the part of those affected by a decision to refuse admission.[2]

The Challenge of HIV/AIDS

The power of illness combined with that to generate arbitrary and emotional responses is nowhere more evident than in state measures to relate control over entry to their territory to HIV. The 'social reality' of fear and prejudice, including the assumption that those affected by HIV are by definition irresponsible and will necessarily engage in anti-social behaviour, more often than not trumps scientific knowledge about transmission and behaviour. Screening and testing are premised on irrational elements in the public health domain (irrational because HIV is not transmitted by casual contact and there is no *inherent* risk); and in the field of costs, because certainly for short-term visitors there is no reason to assume that these will fall on the host community, rather than the country of origin or citizenship.

From an international law and human rights perspective, the issues can be set out quite simply. First, may states, by way of 'blanket exclusions', deny admission to their territory to those with HIV/AIDS, on the grounds of a threat to the public health of the community or liability for health costs? Secondly, may states impose a testing requirement for HIV on all who seek entry? And in either case, what are the limits, if any, imposed by international law and what are the parameters of 'best practice', considered as those policies and procedures which are most conducive to the promotion of state interests and the protection of human rights?

As with most simple questions, the situation in fact is far less straightforward, and the answers considerably more complex and multifaceted. In international law, human rights provide a basis for the control, or moderation, of state powers in the immigration context; to this extent, they reflect recognition of individual rights, entitlements and expectations, many of which will also have community dimensions, in the sense that they contribute to participation and integration in the body politic. State and community interests in public health, in turn, reflect a cluster of related functions, including the assessment of health needs and problems, the development of policies designed to deal with priority health needs, and the adoption of policies and programmes to implement health goals (Gostin and Mann, 1994; Mann *et al.*, 1994). The principle of non-discrimination figures in both contexts, and may be related to a particular working premise, namely, that medical interventions and denial of rights and expectations ought in principle to be based only on a standard of 'significant risk' or its equivalent.

The Spread of Travel Restrictions

Travel advice published by the US Department of State in 1995 indicates that forty-seven states (forty-eight including the USA) now require HIV testing for certain categories of entrants (US Department of State, 1994, 1995). This summary review of state practice reveals considerable diversity, mostly in the length of time for which the potential entrant liable to testing seeks admission, but also by reference to the category of entrant or reason for admission. Some countries require an HIV/AIDS test for anyone intending to remain more than one month; others require that students be tested, or those entering to work. Here some distinguish again, for no apparent reason, on the basis of occupation, singling out hotel staff, hairdressers, entertainers, foreign athletes, or those earning less than a certain wage. Those seeking permanent or extended temporary residence may also be required to submit to testing, although again there is little consistency in either the periods or the exceptions.

Practice, indeed, confirms a mixture of rationality and prejudice. In countries that require testing for those seeking long-term or permanent admission, it may be assumed that the state is committed to the health of the community and therefore also to avoiding additional costs. Where admission for shorter periods is under consideration, the health-related costs argument is less compelling, so far as the individual retains the link of citizenship with his or her own country, and therefore is entitled to receive the care and treatment due in the normal course to all fellow citizens. Testing requirements here appear often to be based on questionable assumptions; for example, relating to the presumed proclivity of the prospective entrant for anti-social or irresponsible conduct: 'entertainers' appear especially subject to suspicion on this account.

The Human Rights Dimension

States retain substantial authority to control the exercise of many human rights, and community membership, including access to citizenship, sits at the centre of the modern notion of the nation-state. Although international law plays a relatively small, direct role in the field of immigration policy, a state's decision to refuse entry, carried out *prima facie* within its area of sovereign competence, may nevertheless have an impact on related rights and interests that require protection. For example, no state may return a refugee to a country in which he or she may be persecuted, or apply measures, such as rejection at the frontier, where the effect is to compel the individual to return to, or remain in, a territory where his or her life, physical integrity or liberty would be threatened for relevant reasons. The 1989 Convention on the Rights of the Child endorses the standard of the 'best interests' of the child which in principle and in appropriate circumstances is capable of prevailing over other considerations, including the legally recognized but competing interests of the state. In a wide range of universal and regional instruments, states have also recognized that the family should receive 'protection by society and the state'; and that 'special measures of protection and assistance should be taken on behalf of all children and young persons'.[3] Together with the principle of the best interests of the child as primary consideration, these considerations put in question any state action with respect to children that might either 'officially' remove the child from the family environment or have the effect of leaving the child without care and support.

Neither the 1951 Convention nor the 1967 Protocol relating to the Status of Refugees deal with health issues, or with the situation of refugees whose admission might raise public health or medical resource questions (UNHCR, 1988). However, sick and disabled refugees certainly figure among 'the most destitute categories' whose admission is called for in UN General

Assembly resolution 428(V), paragraph 2(c), and paragraph 8(d) of the UNHCR Statute; and among those requiring 'permanent custodial care', the 'most needy', and those for whom 'special care' must be provided.[4] With the absence of any formal reference to public health concerns, the essential framework of protection — *non-refoulement* and durable solutions premised on international cooperation and solidarity — nevertheless remains, backed by fundamental principles of human rights.

National and other measures taken to combat AIDS and to prevent the spread of HIV infection can affect every aspect of the refugee's life, from the moment of flight to return home or assimilation in a new national community. They thus need to be related to the objectives established by the international community. For protection purposes, three areas in particular call for attention, namely, screening; the inferences and consequences of testing, particularly in regard to admission, asylum and resettlement; and the treatment of AIDS cases and those who test HIV positive. With respect to screening, it may be assumed in many cases that the ordinary non-national, denied admission because of testing HIV positive, can return to the support system of his or her own community. That possibility is denied to the refugee, for whom *admission, asylum or resettlement* may be the only alternatives to return to persecution. The practice of states in accepting numbers of chronically sick and disabled refugees, including HIV/AIDS cases, shows that humanitarian need can outweigh both fear of costs and risk to the population.

Rights generally must be exercised with due regard to the rights of others; in certain circumstances and within the limits prescribed by international law, governments may restrict their exercise in favour of other community interests. For example, a typical limitation, recognized in similar language in many different treaties, provides with respect to the protected right that, 'No restrictions may be placed on the exercise of this right other than those which are prescribed by law and which are necessary in a democratic society in the interests of national security or public safety, public order (*ordre public*), the protection of public health or morals or the protection of the rights and freedoms of others . . .'[5] States have a margin of appreciation, or discretion, in determining whether and what restrictions may be called for in the light of local circumstances, but the standard of compliance remains an international one. As a general rule, such restrictions are interpreted narrowly, and must be shown to be both necessary and proportional to the end to be achieved. Limitations that exceed what is permissible under international law may be condemned, for example, by decision of a treaty-monitoring mechanism.

Although the right of entry to a state other than one's state of nationality may not be protected *as such* by general international law or human rights treaties, the individual's interest in admission will often be protected indirectly. In a case involving the refusal of admission to the United Kingdom, precisely in a context in which the applicants were not able to invoke a right of entry as such, the European Commission on Human Rights concluded,

'... discrimination based on race could, in certain circumstances of itself amount to degrading treatment within the meaning of Article 3 ... It is generally recognized that a special importance should be attached to discrimination based on race and that publicly to single out a group of persons for differential treatment on the basis of race might ... constitute a special form of affront to human dignity.'[6] The European Commission found that refusal of entry was capable of constituting an interference with the right to respect for family life under Article 8 of the Convention, or of raising a related issue of discrimination. The jurisprudence of European supervisory institutions thus holds considerable precedential value, with a series of consistent rulings in immigration and removal cases that impose significant limitations on sovereign powers.

Non-discrimination and Equal Protection of the Law

Rights such as the right to life, liberty and security of the person and the right to equality before and to the equal protection of the law, clearly allow for no distinction between nationals and aliens. The principle of non-discrimination, originally limited to distinctions drawn on the basis of race alone, has much wider potential today. Unlawful discrimination means some exclusion or restriction, privilege or preference, which has the effect of nullifying a particular right. Those who wish to treat individuals differently must show cause for such differential treatment, and the question in each case is whether the bases advanced for distinction are *relevant*, and thereafter whether the measures adopted are reasonable and proportional.[7] The international legal concept of discrimination thus connotes distinctions which are unfair, unjustifiable or arbitrary.

One question with the principle of non-discrimination is to know precisely where it begins and where it ends. Article 2 of the Universal Declaration of Human Rights provides that 'Everyone is entitled to all the rights and freedoms *set forth in this Declaration*, without distinction of any kind, such as race, colour, sex, language, religion, political or other opinion, national or social origin, property, birth or *other status*'. The UN Sub-Commission on the Prevention of Discrimination and the Protection of Minorities has considered that 'other status' in the non-discrimination context should include health status.[8] Following Article 7 of the Universal Declaration, Article 26 of the 1966 Covenant on Civil and Political Rights provides:

All persons are equal before the law and are entitled without any discrimination to the equal protection of the law. *In this respect*, the law shall prohibit any discrimination and guarantee to all persons equal and effective protection against discrimination on *any ground*

such as race, colour, sex, language, religion, political or other opinion, national or social origin, property, birth or other status.[9]

Equal Treatment and Arbitrary Treatment

Two related issues concern the *rights* sought to be protected, and the *grounds*
on which such rights ought not to be restricted. Specifically, it may be argued
either that international law does not recognize the right to enter a state
other than the state of one's nationality, or that 'health status' is not a relevant basis on which to invoke the principle of non-discrimination. However,
a restriction or limitation that is otherwise permissible must not itself be
imposed in a discriminatory manner, and even though a state may not be
obliged to provide a benefit or entitlement, where it does so then it ought
not to introduce discriminatory measures in its implementation.

In the field of HIV screening for entry, a protected right will be involved, for example, if the applicant falls within the international law provisions on children, the family and refugees. The extent to which such rights
may be restricted is defined with reasonable clarity, and the principle of
equality of treatment may be violated if a distinction is based on a prohibited
ground, including health status, or if it has no objective and reasonable
justification. This in turn will be judged in light of its aim and effects, and
whether there is a reasonable relationship of proportionality between the
means employed and the end sought to be realized.

The refusal of entry on HIV grounds impairs or nullifies the enjoyment
or exercise on an equal footing of rights and freedoms available to others.
Although the right of entry may not be directly at issue, and depending on
the particular circumstances, those rights and freedoms may include the
right of association (for example, with respect to minorities with territorial
homelands covering two or more states), the right to access and to share
information (for example, through participation in international conferences),
the right to education, and the right to employment. As a practical matter,
such civil and political rights may depend for their effective realization on
the movement of persons between states. Each has received a measure of
recognition in international law, and each has the capacity to form the basis
for a (legal and protected) relationship, of one sort or another, between
those who are within and those who are outside the state. It is the task of
international law, drawing on its repertory of norms and principles, to find
a working, workable and equitable balance in the tension between individual
claims/entitlements and state responsibilities.

Notwithstanding the margin of appreciation possessed by states in determining whom to admit to their territory, discrimination on HIV grounds will
be contrary to international law if the aim is 'illegitimate' (which would

include an aim that is illusory or unobtainable), if the means used are disproportionate, and if a protected right or interest is affected. The question whether HIV infection is, in the circumstances, a 'relevant difference' justifying differential treatment must be judged in the light of international standards. The principle of non-discrimination raises a strong presumption of equality, and the party that argues for exceptions must show objective justification and proportionality (Goodwin-Gill, 1978, pp. 58–87). It is not enough to claim that what is in accordance with law and procedure cannot be arbitrary. For it is now generally accepted that an infringement of personal liberty is arbitrary, not only if it is on grounds or in accordance with procedures other than those established by law; but also where it takes place under the provisions of law, the purpose or application of which is incompatible with respect for the right to the integrity, dignity, privacy, liberty or security of the person. What is arbitrary thus embraces what is illegal, but also what is unjust. As the Human Rights Committee has noted with respect to the prohibition against arbitrary interference with family life:[10]

> The expression 'arbitrary interference' . . . can also extend to interference provided for under the law. The introduction of the concept of arbitrariness is intended to guarantee that even interference provided for by law should be in accordance with the provisions, aims and objectives of the Covenant and should be, in any event, reasonable in the particular circumstances.

In principle, exclusion on the basis of HIV infection alone is *prima facie* arbitrary, because it is not related to a public health objective or to a public purse objective. It is premised instead on assumptions with respect to individual behaviour that need to be established on the basis of the facts; and to the mere possibility of a charge on the public purse, which likewise begs proof in the particular case. Similarly, the requirement to submit to screening is likely to be arbitrary in application, so far as it infringes the principle of free and informed consent as a fundamental prerequisite to every intervention, and may leave the applicant without possibility of counselling or treatment.

Screening Policy and the Individuation of Issues

The United States of America is a country that remains committed to immigration and in which debates relating to the criteria for admission and exclusion take place in public. As a country with a high number of people with HIV/AIDS, it must also face some of the longer-term issues, such as community costs. For these reasons, the development of screening policy in the USA in recent years offers considerable insight into the rationale or perceived necessity for exercising control over the entry of those who test HIV positive; at the same time, it helps to identify the sorts of factors that distinguish an arbitrary response from a balanced policy.

From the first broad-sweep restrictions intended to contain the spread of contagious disease, the 1952 Immigration and Nationality Act settled eventually on a policy of excluding persons generally with 'dangerous contagious diseases', and specifically those aliens infected with tuberculosis and leprosy. In 1961, some twenty-one diseases were explicitly identified, but that list had been reduced to seven by 1987: infectious leprosy, active tuberculosis and five sexually transmitted diseases. In that year, legislative changes added HIV to the list of 'dangerous contagious diseases' (Carro, 1989; Starr, 1989;) and a screening programme began, although who was tested depended on the immigration status being sought (Kuntz, 1990). Opposition to screening focused on the fact that it was not an effective control method, and also challenged the assumption that refugees, in particular, were HIV carriers. Moreover, screening failed to deal with key issues, including problems of confidentiality, counselling, refugee protection, effectiveness, public health policy, foreign policy, costs versus benefits to the public, and who should assume responsibility for refugees found to be HIV positive (Keane, 1992).

United States statutory provisions were reviewed during the course of 1990.[11] Scientific evidence and testimony recommended deletion of HIV and all other diseases except infectious tuberculosis, on the ground that they *cannot* be transmitted by 'casual contact, through the air, or from common vehicles such as fomites, food or water'. The governing criterion was in turn changed by the November 1990 Immigration Act, from 'dangerous contagious diseases' to 'communicable diseases of public health significance'. In January 1991, after wide review and reference to external consultants, the Secretary of State for Health and Human Services proposed that only infectious tuberculosis be included as presenting a 'significant public health risk'. The preamble to the proposed new rule noted (McCance, 1992):

> HIV infection is transmitted among adults . . . almost exclusively by two routes: sexual intercourse with an infected person, and the sharing of contaminated injection equipment by injecting drug users. The risk of (or protection from) HIV infection comes not from the nationality of the infected person, but from the specific behaviours that are practised. A careful consideration of epidemiological principles and current medical knowledge leads us to conclude that allowing HIV-infected aliens into this country will not pose a significant additional risk of HIV infection to the US population, where prevalence of HIV infection is already widespread. Our best defence . . . is an educated population.

The period for public comment, however, revealed the extent of the perception that HIV infection was synonymous with extensive health care at tax-payers' expense. The Department of Health and Human Resources' proposal to remove HIV from the list was never adopted; the issue was overtaken by events, and in May 1993 Congress enacted new legislation mandating that 'communicable disease of public health significance' should specifically include 'infection with the etiologic agent for acquired immune deficiency syndrome'.[12]

The legislative aspect, however, is only one part of the picture. Although an immigration applicant infected with HIV is statutorily excludable, waivers continue to be available for the spouse, unmarried son or daughter of a US citizen or non-citizen who has been issued with an immigrant visa; for one who has son or daughter who is a US citizen or permanent resident; for refugees; and for those granted regularization of status under earlier legislation.[13] Temporary visitors also are not routinely tested (*Washington Times*, 1991).

Because HIV-infected applicants are also excludable if likely to become a public charge at any time, a waiver may be obtained by an otherwise eligible applicant who can show that the costs of his or her illness and support will not fall on the public purse. In practice, the Attorney General's discretion will be exercised if the applicant can establish:

1   that the danger to public health through the possible spread of infection created by his or her admission is minimal;
2   that the possibility of the spread of infection as a result of his or her admission also is minimal; and
3   that no cost will be incurred by any US government agency without prior consent of that agency.

The 'individualization' of the exercise of discretion is illustrated by reference to the type of evidence generally required, including the fact that the applicant has arranged for medical treatment in the United States, that he or she is aware of the nature and severity of the medical condition, is willing to attend education seminars and counselling sessions, and knows of the modes of transmission of the disease.[14] Moreover, in determining the question of likelihood to become a public charge, relevant factors will include an offer of employment in the United States, the applicant's ability to undertake the employment, his or her own financial resources and/or those of family members, the availability of adequate and affordable medical insurance, and ability to meet living costs.

Conclusion

The World Health Organization has long maintained that HIV/AIDS constitutes no threat to public health. HIV infection is not like certain psychopathic conditions in which the afflicted are *unable* to control their behaviour and for that reason constitute a potential danger to other members of society. Similarly, HIV infection is not like infectious conditions, such as tuberculosis, in which regardless of the best efforts of the person affected, others are likely to be put at risk, for example, through airborne transmission of bacteria. Although there is no hard evidence to suggest that HIV/AIDS-related costs justify travel restrictions, the perceptions among legislators and administrators are to the contrary; barriers to travel appear to be increasing, not only with respect to those seeking to migrate permanently, but also for those travelling to work or to study.

In this context, HIV screening appears to serve two functions, neither of which is dictated by health or economics. From the perspective of an uninformed and apprehensive public, for whom elected representatives want to be seen to be 'doing something', screening seems an easy enough and necessary way by which to raise a barrier to the spread of disease and to protect the public purse. In fact, its limitations with respect to the prevention of transmission of HIV are common knowledge, including the 'window of uncertainty' between possible infection and the development of antibodies, and the notorious reluctance on the part of states to test citizens returning from abroad, even from 'high risk' areas. But there are other problems with any screening programme, including the suspicion engendered, the temptation to report inexact medical histories, or to breach confidentiality, and the practical difficulties of follow-up where appropriate (Loutan, 1992). As one commentator has remarked, countries requiring HIV testing commonly accept refugees for resettlement having medical conditions likely to incur public expense far in excess of anything an HIV patient is likely to incur, and this rather negates the argument for screening on economic grounds (Keane, 1992).

Applicable International Human Rights Standards

Recognized human rights may be extensively affected by policies of screening and travel restrictions, even though the right of entry to a foreign state, as such, is not protected. The principle of non-discrimination shows how singling out a particular group for differential treatment, such as those who are or are believed to be HIV-positive, may violate their rights. Compulsory testing jeopardizes the integrity of the individual, contravening the principle of 'free and informed consent' as the most fundamental requirement for any medical intervention.[15] In certain circumstances, to test individuals without also offering the possibility of treatment or counselling will likely constitute cruel or inhuman or degrading treatment, especially if such testing is not necessary, is not related to a legitimate objective, or is out of proportion to the aim sought to be realized.

In much the same way, the Council of Europe's draft bioethics convention would restrict tests predictive of genetic diseases to 'health purposes' or 'research linked to health purposes'.[16] Among the complicating factors noted in the draft explanatory memorandum are the fact that such testing 'generates information not only on the individual concerned, but also on future offspring and biologically related family members. The right to privacy thus involves more than one individual and calls for particular attention'.[17] Further complications arise in the case of predictive testing, where there is *at present no treatment available*: 'In such diseases, screening should remain exceptional . . . It would put too much strain on the free participation and on the privacy of individuals'.[18]

Determinations of admissibility in the immigration context, to conform with principle, ought therefore to be taken solely on the basis of information relating to the personal circumstances of the individual, not on the basis of assumptions having no scientific or other equivalent foundation. For example, it cannot be assumed, with respect to a non-immigrant otherwise 'returnable' to his or her country of origin/citizenship, that HIV infection, or even AIDS, makes it likely that he or she will become a public charge in the state contemplating admission. The principle against arbitrariness, coupled with principles of respect for human dignity, privacy and integrity, non-discrimination and equality before the law, requires further that the fact of HIV infection should not raise a presumption that the individual in question will engage in anti-social behaviour (that is, conduct likely to lead to the spread of the virus).

HIV-based travel restrictions have a serious impact on the rights, interests and expectations of individuals, families and communities. In order to take account of those rights and interests, many of which are clearly recognized by international law and in the practice of states, as well as of the sovereign concerns of states themselves, restrictions ought only to be imposed on the basis of a finding of significant risk to the community of the state contemplating admission; that is, in order to avert *probable* harm to the health or safety of others.[19] A similar standard ought to apply to the question of costs, bearing in mind the circumstances of the individual, continuing links to the country of origin/citizenship, and the corresponding benefits to be gained from admission, for example, through the labour or other contribution of the applicant for entry.

Case Assessment Standards

From a practical point of view, the objectives of principle set out above are only likely to be achieved by way of policies and procedures that adhere generally to another principle common to most legal and administrative systems, namely, that of rationally justified decisions; this means that decisions ought to be reasoned by reference to rational objectives, and justified by reference to individual circumstances.

In the case of decisions on the admission to state territory of non-citizens with HIV/AIDS, the rational objectives endorsed in the practice of states include protecting the public health of the community, and protecting the public purse from excessive demands on health services. Whether an individual constitutes a risk to public health, for example, on the basis of actual or likely behaviour, is evidently a question to be answered in the light of his or her personal circumstances. Equally, the possibility that he or she will incur costs to the receiving community will depend on the nature or length of anticipated stay, personal arrangements, such as insurance or employment, and the existence of family or other support. The context in which such decisions are taken, however, is potentially replete with competing rights and interests, many of which are firmly based in international human rights law.

Whatever general policy is adopted, international standards are most likely to be met where individuals are personally interviewed; where potential elements justifying denial of admission are evaluated clearly; and where decisions are based on the available evidence. 'Best practice' will therefore allow the individual to show that the risk to public health through the possible spread of infection created by admission is minimal, for example, because he or she is aware of the nature and severity of the medical condition; knows how it is transmitted and how its spread may be prevented; has arranged for treatment and counselling; and is prepared to act responsibly.

With respect to the likelihood of costs to the public, the individuated approach allows the applicant for entry to show that any expense will not fall upon the community, for example because he or she is able to undertake employment, and has access to financial resources, including insurance or support from family or community organizations, which will ensure medical treatment and an adequate standard of living.

Finally, a higher standard of protection of children and refugees, due under international law by reason of their particularly vulnerable situation or the loss of national community, will require dispensation from certain restrictive provisions. 'Best practice' therefore should provide for discretion to admit children and refugees, where the humanitarian and compassionate equities outweigh conflicting interests, and even in circumstances in which the host community must bear support costs.

Notes

1   This paper draws extensively on the author's work for the World Health Organization during 1995. The author is grateful for the extensive assistance and advice

provided during that time by Dr Doris Schopper, Chief, a.i., Planning, Policy and Co-operation, and Susan Timberlake, Human Rights Officer, WHO Global Programme on AIDS. The views expressed, however, are those of the author, and are not necessarily shared by WHO or the United Nations.

2   See Article 4(1) and Annex, which in turn prescribes as diseases which might endanger public health, those subject to quarantine listed in International Health Regulation No. 2 of the World Health Organization of 25 May 1951; tuberculosis of the respiratory system in an active state or showing a tendency to develop; syphilis; and other infectious diseases of contagious parasitic diseases if the subject of provisions for the protection of nationals of the host country. See also Directive 72/194/EEC, 18 May 1972.

3   Article 23(1), 1966 Covenant on Civil and Political Rights; and Article 10(3), 1966 Covenant on Economic, Social and Cultural Rights, respectively.

4   UNGA resolutions 430(V), 14 December 1950, 639(VII), 20 December 1952 and 728(VIII), 23 October 1953.

5   See for example Article 22(1), 1966 Covenant on Civil and Political Rights.

6   S.M.L. Patel (Application No. 4403/70) and others v. UK, Decision of the European Commission of Human Rights, October 1970, *Collection of Decisions*, **32**, p. 92.

7   Cf. Judge Tanaka, *South West Africa Cases* (Second Phase), ICJ *Reports*, 1966, **6**, 305f, 313.

8   UN doc. E/CN.4/Sub.2/1994/L.42.

9   See also Article 24, 1969 American Convention on Human Rights.

10   Human Rights Committee, General Comments, No. 16, § 4: UN doc. CCPR/C/21/Rev.1, 19 May 1989 (emphasis supplied).

11   Controversy was aroused by the detention in 1989 of a Dutch non-immigrant seeking to attend an international AIDS conference in the United States. Several international organizations protested by boycotting the following year's AIDS conference in San Francisco. A special ten-day visa was created for those attending certain conferences, which did not require applicants to state if they were HIV positive; see *Interpreter Releases*, **72**, p. 1338 (2 October 1995), note 5 and text.

12   National Institutes of Health Revitalization Act 1993, amending section 212(a)(1)(A)(i) of the Immigration and Nationality Act; see 139 *Congressional Record*, No. 17, 18 February 1993, S1762 (in which health costs and the health of Americans were mentioned as factors justifying the legislation); also *Interpreter Releases*, **70**, p. 349 (22 March 1993); p. 677 (24 May 1993).

13   INA, section 212(g); *Interpreter Releases*, **72**, p. 1338 (2 October 1995).

14   'Immigrant Waivers for Aliens found Excludable under Section 212(a)(1)A(i) of the Immigration and Nationality Act due to HIV Infection', Memorandum dated 6 September 1995, by T. Alexander Aleinikoff, Executive Associate Commissioner for Programs; text in *Interpreter Releases*, **72**, p. 1347 (2 October 1995).

15   Council of Europe Draft Convention, Articles 2, 5.

16   *Ibid*, Article 17.

17   *Ibid*, Draft Explanatory Memorandum, para. 113.

18   *Ibid*, para. 114.
19   The simple invocation of public health grounds, therefore, would not suffice to establish risk to the community.

References

ALSTON, P. (Ed.) (1992) *The United Nations and Human Rights*, Clarendon Press: Oxford.

CARRO, J.L. (1989) 'From constitutional psychopathic inferiority to AIDS: What is in the future for homosexual aliens?', *Yale Law and Policy Review*, **7**, pp. 201.

CASTLES, S., BOOTH, H. and WALLACE, T. (1984) *Here for Good*, London: Pluto Books.

COUNCIL OF EUROPE (1994) Draft Convention for the Protection of Human Rights and Dignity of the Human Being with Regard to the Application of Biology and Medicine Bioethics Convention, CE Doc. 7124, 11 July.

GOODWIN-GILL, G.S. (1978) *International Law and the Movement of Persons between States*, Oxford: Clarendon Press, pp. 58–87.

GOODWIN-GILL, G.S. (1996) *The Refugee in International Law*, 2nd edn, Oxford: Clarendon Press.

GOSTIN, L. and MANN, J.M. (1994) 'Towards the development of a human rights impact assessment for the formulation and evaluation of public health policy', *Health and Human Rights*, **1**, p. 59.

HAMMAR, T. (1985) *European Immigration Policy*, Cambridge: Cambridge University Press.

KEANE, V. (1992) 'Migrant medical screening: A confusing blend', *International Migration*, **30**, pp. 209–11.

KUNTZ, D. (1990) 'Contagious disease and refugee protection: AIDS policy in the United States,' *International Migration*, **28**, pp. 379–81.

LOUTAN, L. (1992) 'Medical screening of asylum seekers in Switzerland', *International Migration*, **30**, pp. 223–30.

MANN, J.M., GOSTIN, L., GRUSKIN, S., BRENNAN, T., LAZZARINI, Z. and FINEBERG, H.V. (1994) 'Health and human rights', in BAGNOUD, F.-X. (Ed.) *Health and Human Rights*, **1**, p. 7.

McCANCE, C. (1992) 'Medical screening of migrants: Current national requirements in the United States', *International Migration*, **30**, pp. 215–19.

PLENDER, R. (1988) *International Migration Law*, 2nd edn, Dordrecht: Nijhoff.

SIEGHART, P. (1983) *The International Law of Human Rights*, Oxford: Clarendon Press.

STARR, P. (1989) 'The ineffectiveness and impact of the human immunodeficiency virus (HIV) exclusion in US immigration law', *Geo. Imm. L.J.*, **3**, 87.

UNITED NATIONS (1945) CHARTER ARTICLES 2(1), 2(4) and 2(7).

UNITED NATIONS HIGH COMMISSIONER FOR REFUGEES (1988) 'Policy and guidelines regarding refugee protection and assistance and acquired immune deficiency syndrome (AIDS)', UNHCR/IOM/21/88-UNHCR/FOM/20/88, 15 Feb. 1988.

UNITED STATES DEPARTMENT OF STATE, BUREAU OF CONSULAR AFFAIRS (1994) 'Human immunodeficiency virus (HIV): Testing requirements for entry into foreign countries', December 1994, updated March 1995.

WASHINGTON TIMES, 21 February 1991, cited by Legomsky, S.H. (1992) *Immigration Law and Practice*, Oxford: Clarendon Press.

Chapter 5

The Person Behind the Virus:
Migration, Human Factors and Some Moral and Ethical Questions

Lorraine Sherr and Calliope Farsides

Migration is the global term referring to movement. It is a concept enshrined into the understanding and unravelling of the HIV epidemic and one which carries with it political, ethical, psychological, social and medical ramifications. Although there is a clear legal definition of migration, any analysis of the ethical impact of movement must also be conceptualized at other levels to provide a comprehensive picture of the triggers to movement, the reactions to movement and the constraints on movement. Movements across state borders are traditionally the domain of migration, but there are other subtle forms of movement, within states and between states, which have bearing on the HIV debate.

Migration has the potential to become an ethical problem even before one introduces the complicating factor of HIV. Essentially the problems arise when restrictions are placed upon migration, either by states refusing their citizens the right to leave, or by would-be migrants being refused entry to their chosen destination. In both cases a fundamental human right to freedom of movement would appear to have been thwarted, but we need to ask further questions before stating that this is unjustifiable.

In the first case the issue might appear clear cut — citizens should be allowed to leave their home state, especially if another country is happy to receive them. However, we might feel that some citizens have an obligation to remain within a country in return for benefits they have gained. For example, if someone has been supported through an expensive medical education it might be felt that they should spend a minimum period working within their own country before venturing elsewhere. In the second case, the issues are far more complex. In some situations we regard movement across borders as positively advantageous, and encourage it, as in the European Community's drive towards a mobile European workforce, or where traditional and lucrative trade routes have crossed national borders.

In the early days of the HIV epidemic it was sometimes possible to isolate sources of HIV infection. In the quest for understanding the cause of this disease, disproportionate attention was, and still may be, focused on the source group when, and if, it is easily identified. Discrimination and outgroup labelling emerge as an obvious hazard. HIV was often described in terms of cross border travel (Vittecoq *et al.*, 1987) in the early accounts and conceptualized as an 'imported problem' (Gilmore *et al.*, 1989). As HIV infection moves to a worldwide pandemic, there is often a clear pattern which can be discerned in the way the epidemic moves within a country. Early infection is often typified as outsider infection. As cases then arise within isolated groups, the concept moves to 'insider outsiders'. This refers to other groups, often outgroups, who are then easily blamed for the epidemic such as 'gay men', 'drug (ab)users', 'refugees', people with haemophilia — indeed anyone other than the self. The direct danger of these approaches is the ease with which societies are able to label such outsiders in order to avoid taking action. The inevitable move of the virus into the wider community often triggers a reaction of restriction of movement in an attempt to restrict the spread of the virus (Gostin *et al.*, 1990). Very often the subtle implication of such a strategy, be it overt or covert, is to attack the people with the virus, rather than the virus itself.

People move for all kinds of reasons. This movement often mirrors the course of the epidemic of HIV (Quinn, 1994). Some causes of movement are external to HIV, triggered by economic, community or social factors. However, as time progresses and the epidemic unwinds, some movement patterns are more directly linked to HIV itself. Examples of such trails can be seen with truck drivers in Africa, sex workers in Thailand, and injecting drug users in Scotland. The ethical questions raised concern the rights of such movement as well as the logic, if any, of restricting such movement. Any analysis of rights of movement must be supplemented by an analysis of other more subtle forms of movement present in the HIV arena. For example, can treatments move? Can medical procedures migrate and travel? If they do, on what basis should such movement occur, and what restrictions and restraints should be applied? The argument can extend to products, with an interesting example posed by products which have been implicated in HIV transmission, such as blood products, as well as by semen donation.

This chapter will briefly consider some of the many challenges posed by migration, HIV, and the psychology of some of the underpinning ethical and moral questions they raise, exploring a selected few of the many possible examples which could be raised.

Migration as a Risk for HIV

HIV infection has been monitored as it spreads across trade routes in east Africa (Carswell *et al.*, 1989; Wawer *et al.*, 1991) or along highways in rural India

(Singh and Malavivya, 1994). Urban prevalence is often noted as higher than rural (Barongo *et al.*, 1992), with an intermediate prevalence noted in systematic samples of roadside settlements. Plummer *et al.* (1991) report that a study of long-distance truck drivers revealed that 61 per cent had contact with sex workers, with 25 per cent visiting a prostitute at least weekly. It seems that behaviours that may enhance HIV exposure may also be associated with migrant work. Any analysis of such behavioural patterns needs to address the social and economic factors preceding such behaviour, such as those contributing to a situation where women involved in sex work have few other means of livelihood and where there is also a large migrant male labour force.

Many travel restrictions originate ostensibly in the belief that migration itself poses a risk of HIV transmission. Whilst the logic of this belief needs to be fully explored, at the same time the indirect effects of restrictions may be associated with the further transmission it sets out to avoid. The risk is not simply migration, but the behaviour of individuals who may or may not be migrants. Such restrictions also often overlook short-term back and forth travel which is not only extensive, but growing (Hawkes *et al.*, 1994). Migration patterns in many African cities, for example, have provided conditions which are said to enhance HIV transmission. If migration affects social circumstances, interventions for change can be focused at root causes, social consequences, or the migration itself. It is distressing to note how often the former two are overlooked, while focus is maintained on the migration.

Among forms of population movement that may be linked to HIV, one as yet neglected is that of runaway youth. Stricof *et al.* (1991) showed a high HIV prevalence of 5.3 per cent in a survey carried out in a facility for run-away youth in the US. Allen *et al.* (1994) extended such an analysis to fourteen US cities and confirmed these findings. One of the problems in interpreting these data may be a failure to accept that HIV itself may make people run away or become homeless if discrimination, unemployment and enforced homelessness result from revelations of HIV status. Gutman (1994) points out that young people who run away are usually desperate, without support or protection and are poorly prepared to ensure a safe life, with common recourse to sexual favours, prostitution and drug-related activities; all of which may enhance exposure to HIV. It is unclear whether risk activity results from homelessness or in homelessness. The problem is a growing one and to date it is clear that among these groups HIV prevalence is high, but the causes and interventions need careful examination.

Furthermore, migration not only marks movement, but also marks separation. The separation (rather than the migration) may itself account for increased exposure to risk situations and risk behaviour. Along similar lines, Ryder *et al.* (1990) and Wilkins *et al.* (1991) noted an increased prevalence of HIV in divorced or separated individuals. However, it would be difficult to make any ethical conclusions as it is unclear whether divorced/separated individuals go on to have more partners or whether the opposite is true: i.e. people who have more partners have a greater tendency to divorce or separate.

Control of Movement

Most countries have created a legal structure in order to contain or control population movement. With any form of control the underlying philosophy for the reason of control must be analysed. It is at this juncture that the needs of the individual and society may need to be compared. In many countries control over movement on the basis of HIV status has been instituted and the justification of this must be questioned.

At a general level, although a national government has primary responsibility for the welfare of its own citizens, nations also have responsibilities and obligations towards one another and this might sometimes entail offering refuge to members of a country which cannot support its own people. Furthermore, when a country abuses its own people or subjects them to war, we as global citizens should feel some responsibility to protect them. Thus we generally make a special case for refugees and asylum seekers when deciding whether or not immigration should be allowed.

Having said this it is difficult to argue that a country has an obligation to welcome in anyone and everyone who wishes to reside in it. It may be necessary to limit the level of immigration into a country for a number of reasons, and it may sometimes be necessary to prevent specific individuals entering. But, given that in doing so we prevent an individual moving freely and thus restrict a fundamental liberty, we need a strong justification. If it were the case that a high level of immigration were to put a strain on already stretched resources, thus seriously threatening the well-being of the resident population, a government might well feel justified in putting the needs of its own people first.

Let us assume for the moment, however, that the political situation in state X, a poor developing country state, is such that a minority group within the population are in real danger of being persecuted and ultimately killed if they remain. Few could deny that by standard criteria those affected should be allowed to enter country Y, a more prosperous developed country, as refugees. Furthermore, the numbers in question are certainly not high enough to trigger arguments against their entry on the basis of threats to the well-being of the host country. If there is known to be a fairly high prevalence of HIV infection in state X, the question is whether this should have any bearing on who is granted entry. The argument should surely go something like this. Certain individuals from state X have a special need to enter state Y as political refugees. This need is formally recognized and state Y will accept as many refugees as it can without posing a serious threat to the well-being of its own citizens. The fact that any one of these individual refugees may be HIV positive is only relevant if this in itself is thought to pose a serious threat. There appear to be two potential threats of harm related to the refugees being HIV positive. First, they may infect others once within the host country. Second, they may place an intolerable strain on the host country's medical and social service resources. Both these points can be dealt with quite successfully.

Having said this there would appear to be no reason to refuse a person who otherwise has a claim to entry because they are HIV positive. Nor is there any need to test refugees on entry (see discussion of the Ethiopian Jews, below). To do so would effectively be a form of discrimination and may entail coercion, with people feeling forced to comply with testing for fear of being refused entry or subsequent support. If no argument has been offered to support testing of the general population, it is difficult to support the idea of testing a section of the population just because of the HIV prevalence in their country of origin. This is not to say that individuals could not be counselled and allowed to choose for themselves whether or not to be tested.

However, being liberal on this issue might cause its own problems. What happens in practice is that, in the absence of knowledge about a particular individual's status, judgments may be made about the individual on the basis of the known or presumed prevalence of the virus within the group to which he or she belongs. If it is well known that HIV/AIDS is a serious problem in state X all refugees might find themselves treated as if they were HIV positive themselves. Where discriminative practice exists, this could have detrimental effects on the individual.

In the US, immigration controls in connection with HIV were introduced in 1987 (Fairchild and Tynan, 1994). The rulings on which this was based, however, differentiated between short- and long-term movement, namely immigration and holidays. It provided an odd distinction on public health grounds, given that any 'risky behaviour' could obviously be carried out in a short- or long-term stay. Thus it was not necessarily exposure to an individual at any given occasion with HIV, but more about arbitrary longer-term movement or perhaps the cost implications that illness may have on the broader society. If this was indeed true, one would expect a more sensible and sensitive provision which may provide for waivers according to means, ability to self-fund care or illness parameters. No such waivers were obvious.

Whenever migration or movement restrictions are brought into force within a country, they are invariably accompanied by a multitude of allied problems relating to the implementation and logistics of such rulings. Immigration control has not been shown to succeed as an HIV prevention measure despite the fact that some countries still opt for it. Extremes can be seen in countries such as Sweden where there is provision for isolation and incarceration to be utilized as an option. Social isolation can also make the situation difficult, as, for example, has been seen in Japan (Hoshino, 1995). The lessons from abortion and prohibition have been overlooked: such measures rarely stop the activity, but inevitably result in loss of control, its movement underground, exploitation and corruption.

Freedom to Cross Borders

Guidelines about freedoms such as that to cross borders need to be pondered. Is there ever any moral right to refuse entry to an HIV positive individual? This raises an old question of whether toleration of the intolerant is morally, ethically or legally defensible.

Freedom of movement raises complex moral questions. The initial question is that of competing rights. Erin (1995) points out that the rights to remain in a country may be greater than the rights of entry to that country. This immediately brings into being an analysis of individuals into different categories in terms of their freedoms and rights. In reality the richer, privileged societies close their borders and present restrictions to the poorer. Where do the ethics of entry refusal lie in terms of corresponding obligations? For example, if you fail to allow nationals into a country to better their condition, is there a duty to attempt to help them improve their situation in their own country?

Refusal of Entry

HIV restrictions may extend to refusal of entry to a country. To understand why states may make such refusals, it is important to explore the real reasons that may underlie the stated reasons. Grounds of public health are often invoked to rationalize and justify contraint and restrictions. For a variety of reasons, this may be an untenable argument with HIV and AIDS. Those who invoke public health arguments for exclusion essentially claim that by keeping infection out of a state, one can be taking steps to ensure the future health of the nationals of that state. Although simplistic and appearing straightforward, this is not really the case with HIV when the practicalities are explored. The state would need to simultaneously restrict movement of its nationals outside of its borders. If a state is protecting the uninfected, is there a corresponding possibility that the state would then attempt to expel all its own existing nationals who test HIV positive? To do that would then require regular monitoring of HIV status, and even if this was carried out (the logistics of which would probably render it impossible), it would miss the newly infected who may be seroconverting and include all false positives. The expulsion of citizens is not theoretically impossible based on this line of argument. If a state asserts a public health morality, why is this morality confined to their own public? Why is it that no state has contemplated refusing exit to HIV positive individuals in order to reduce infectivity elsewhere, and only refusal of entry is contemplated? Surely the protection of other nationals is equally ethically justified if the premise is to hold at all (Harris,

1995). Harris (1995) further points out that some people are in the dynamic process of becoming citizens and ethical/moral behaviour should apply to a citizen seeker as well as a citizen. Indeed if unethical restrictions are visited on citizen seekers, do they have redress if and when they become citizens?

Reasons for Control

The reasons for control over migration in relation to HIV can be many, including financial (to limit health care costs or preserve health care resources), to protect citizens or the public health, or because of discrimination. Often control is an ill-thought-out first-line reaction to an insoluble problem. In many countries without clearly articulated policies and procedures, an initial attempt to be active includes promotion of HIV testing in the belief, however inaccurate, that this may in some way divert the problem. Such policies often wreak havoc and misery, rarely prevent new infection, and often create a counterproductive milieu of fear, distrust and avoidance.

When the testing of migrants is not clearly thought through, the long-term problems that are raised can be enormous. For example in 1991, 19 000 Ethiopian Jews were airlifted to Israel. On arrival the authorities decided to screen all for HIV with no mention of pre-test counselling and not with the intention of refusing entry. Thus it is unclear what purpose testing was intended to serve. The entire procedure raised enormous problems with confidentiality. Furthermore it also suggested arbitrary discrimination given that other immigrants, say from the US and the USSR, were not screened in the same way. Case management, planning and policy were limited or non-existent, resulting in chaos, isolation, rejection and much blame of those who were HIV positive on arrival (Shtarkshall, 1995).

Enforcing Restrictions

In order realistically to enforce restrictions based on HIV status, one has to have a service in place which can establish HIV status — categorically — in the first instance. This may then raise a controversy surrounding how HIV testing of potential migrants is carried out, who does the test, whose standard is acceptable, and whether individuals need to be tested in their country of origin or country of arrival. Theoretically this brings with it a host of problems associated with the procedures required in order to gain a blood sample. What would happen, say, if an individual is exposed to a dirty needle because of HIV testing? If they were infected by the very procedure which was set to establish their negativity could there be some liability?

Of course this is all based on the presumption of perfect procedure — a background which is in fact incorrect. The HIV test itself is not perfect. Indeed the very nature of its imperfection may dramatically affect its implementation. Any test without perfect sensitivity or specificity may give false negatives and false positives. The HIV antibody test cannot detect antibodies during the early weeks of infection while the body is still mounting an antibody reaction. During this window of time, not only can the test come back negative despite the individual being infected, but the individual is at heightened infectivity. If a false negative result is given to an individual who is in fact HIV positive, is there any liability if subsequent risk exposure results from the inaccurate reassurance?

The more 'liberal' countries, which do not place restrictions, still perpetrate some of the outsider notions in the way they gather data. For example Hawkes *et al.* (1994) report that 'since 1984, 63 per cent of heterosexually acquired HIV infections reported within the United Kingdom to the CDSC have been in people who either lived in or visited WHO Pattern II countries'. Data covering HIV infection in people who originate outside a country and/ or have had sexual exposure or even travel abroad is routinely collected and reported in countries such as the UK (Noone *et al.*, 1991; Communicable Disease Report, 1992), Belgium (Bonneux *et al.*, 1988) and Holland (Houweling and Coutinho, 1991), and also amongst European drug users (Richardson *et al.*, 1993). Therein lies a presumption that the exposure must have come from abroad, given that no data is reported on sexual or other risks while 'at home'. The scenario provided means that anyone who has had sex abroad is at a differential risk than someone who has had sex in their home country, irrespective of the safety, nature or frequency of such acts. The conclusions are also problematic in that there is a presumption that it was the act abroad that was associated with the infection rather than acts at home. Studies on travellers (e.g. Hawkes *et al.*, 1994) examine sexual behaviour abroad, yet few give details of sexual behaviour at home. There is some evidence to suggest that behaviour at home and away may vary, indeed that the point of the trip was sexually motivated, but there may well be an argument that those who seek out risky sexual experience abroad may also do so within the borders of their home country (one fifth in the Hawkes study had been treated for STDs in the past five years — perhaps an indication of their sexual behaviour).

Asylum Seeking and Refugees

Many countries where HIV is endemic are also experiencing war and unrest. As a result there may be refugee communities domiciled or attempting to reside in safer centres. Such refugees bring with them large burdens of particular problems, and HIV may often be peripheral to their predicament. The ethical questions raised are often enormous. For instance, there is the dilemma of divulging HIV status when it is feared that such status may jeopardize the according of legal status as a refugee: some asylum seekers who are concerned about their status may not seek out appropriate medical care for fear of jeopardizing their acceptance into a country. Discrimination, a hazard associated with refugee status, is exacerbated by HIV issues.

The specific group of people seeking asylum may include those whose triggers include the effects of discrimination, maltreatment or lack of public health measures relating to AIDS and HIV. The problems such individuals face is the overt or covert nature of such suffering. Should they let it be known that this is the basis on which they seek asylum and would this, in turn, jeopardize or enhance their chances of success? Is there an ethical basis for seeking asylum based on the lack of provision for HIV-related conditions? It is unclear, again, whether the basis of such responses are founded in human rights, acceptance of human suffering, or the more subtle motivations such as finance. If reciprocal treatment agreements were in place, would this obviate the need to have border restrictions?

HIV as a Risk for Migration

On the other hand there is a case that HIV infection may trigger movement. This may be directly as a result of discrimination or stigma. For example, people with HIV infection may move to centres of excellence to ensure quality care and up-to-date treatment, to protect themselves from health care workers who may be prejudiced or unwilling to provide them with high quality care, or for reasons of confidentiality.

Indirectly, movement may result when communities break down because of high prevalence of HIV disease. The death of parents is an example where AIDS may trigger movement of children either to grandparents or to extended family for care, or to the city in order to establish self-sufficiency. A major problem associated with the concepts of restriction, control and eradication is one of short-sighted reaction. Education, prevention and resources need to be provided for such recently arrived groups — yet this is overlooked. In a study by Oppenheim (1994), fifty-four newly migrated individuals were studied when they presented at service agencies. Of these, thirteen reported needle-sharing for the administration of medication, and only one had access to non-emergency medical care. This study clearly points out the dangers of marginalizing new immigrants as a possible risk activity on the part of the host state.

Movement and the Military

Military data is often not explored thoroughly in terms of its potential role in HIV transmission. This is odd, given that many studies look for seroprevalence in military recruits and then fail to monitor their sexual behaviour as they move, or do not proceed to provide health education after HIV testing. This is worrying, given that large numbers of HIV positive people are identified in such studies. Cowan *et al.* (1994) report that the overall infection incidence rates among soldiers in active and reserve components of the US army are similar (.25 per 1 000 per year). Additionally, studies which explore risk are often one-sided. For example Garland *et al.* (1993) examined the association between HIV seroconversion with visits to foreign ports of US navy personnel. They noted 813 seroconverters but found no increased risk of seroconversion due to visits to foreign ports. However, the study did not deem it necessary to study the possible infection of foreign nationals at these ports by the HIV positive naval personnel.

Duties and Obligations

There is an entire debate which needs to consider where duty ends and where moral obligations end. There is a growing school of thought which attempts to explore HIV issues in relation to the rights and responsibilities debate. This debate sets up a corresponding social contract where rights need to be appreciated not for their own merit, but within a reciprocal framework of corresponding responsibilities. This is often explored in terms of safe sex, infection and culpability for infecting others. The hidden notions underlying this debate raise many problems. For example, the debate may claim that individuals with HIV may only have rights to move and travel to a country if they undertake reciprocal obligations not to infect others whilst in that country. Such an argument may have a surface appeal, but it overlooks the two-way nature of infection, namely that unsafe sex requires more than one partner. It also does not account for acts such as rape and abuse.

The Individual and the Community

Kirby (1989) has eloquently articulated the tension between individual and community rights where the freedom of the individual becomes questioned at the point that it contacts or indeed conflicts with the self-same freedoms and rights of others. This concept can be examined in terms of migration. Does this imply that the good of the whole community has an overriding effect on the rights of the individual? Policies need to be developed so that the rights of the individual and those of the society can both be accommodated without setting them against each other. If the individual is perceived as part of the community, rather than in conflict with it, this is more likely to occur. In practice, compassion usually works more effectively than repression and restraint. Policy must be formulated prior to the event, with carefully thought out, articulated, argued and resourced strategies, rather than reactive measures which are often short-sighted, limited in focus and reactionary.

Vulnerable Groups

In Europe there may well be a situation where vulnerable groups have a disproportionate burden of HIV in their communities. This may result from a number of factors. There may well be an accumulation of vulnerability which exacerbates the situation. Such groups can be identified among drug users, children, refugee communities, women, the underprivileged or the poor. These categories are not necessarily mutually exclusive, and many problems occur when they exist in tandem. There is then an ethical challenge to protect groups who are vulnerable. Could one make the argument that the migration of those unable to look after themselves adequately should be helped to a greater extent than those who are? Are there principles of social justice which need to be examined in the way the HIV epidemic unfolds? There are certainly arguments that groups that are disenfranchised, poor and discriminated against have the right to protection. The distribution of power and political muscle to enact policy is such that the disenfranchised need to rely on the good will and benevolence of those in power in order to have their voices heard.

Movement of Ideas

Control is often viewed in terms of the movement of people. However, one can expand some of the moral and ethical issues to a wider range of movement. For example the movement of research is one which has been of notable proportion in the field of HIV.

For a variety of reasons, research on this disease is often carried out by the nationals of one country on the nationals of another. The arguments for this are varied, ranging from philanthropic (provide high tech to the poor), through colonization (establishing a research base in another country), or mutual need (gather data from centres where prevalence is high to inform parts of the world where it is still low). Sadly, in reality high prevalence is concentrated in poorer countries, and thus there is a potential moral and ethical problem where the well-to-do countries export research, clinical trials, procedures or medication interventions to areas other than their own to gather publications, scientific knowledge or insight for the benefit of those in their country. What are the rules governing such circumstances? For example should the principals behind such interventions ensure that standards are at least the same as for their own nationals? This is all well and good if such standards are acceptable, but in reality the situation may be complex. Take for example a study to promote condom use. If the safety standard for condoms in one country requires a very high price per unit, could this standard morally and ethically be compromised in order to allow a study which would permit free distribution of condoms in a poorer centre? Could there ever be grounds to use the cheaper product (with the higher breakage rates) if the alternative was that there were no condoms available?

For some questions, it is impossible to perform studies in centres where the funding may well be available simply because there are not enough cases available. Take for example the possibility that Caesarean section may reduce vertical transmission of HIV from mother to baby. Findings from European studies are equivocal, and the studies themselves methodologically weak since the women in them were not randomly allocated to the procedure. In the absence of good research findings, clinical practice may be to advocate Caesarean section anyway. This may have a number of costs which are counter-productive on medical (Semprini *et al.*, 1995) and psychological grounds (Sherr, 1995) and certainly one could argue that good research is needed to guide clinical practice and decision-making for women. Such data could be provided if 1 500 women could be randomly allocated to Caesarean section versus vaginal delivery (Newell, 1995), a figure far in excess of the deliveries of HIV positive women in any single European country. The study would need to recruit samples from areas of higher prevalence, such as South Africa, and it is here that the ethical and moral questions come into play. If, for the best of reasons, women from the developing world are recruited into a study to test the efficacy of an invasive surgical procedure on vertical transmission outcome, what are the moral constraints on the migration of such research? Should the same medical benefits in the European centres be available to the women in the developing centre? Should there be financial compensation? Should such procedures only be exported with guarantees that if they are proved to be efficacious they would then be available in the developing country? How is informed consent sought and do the same professional patient norms operate in both centres? If not, what steps ought to be taken in order to harmonize them?

Which Way Forward?

Migration challenges very basic notions of rights, discrimination and moral behaviour in the way any culture or society responds to HIV infection. People are subject to the restrictions and ramifications of policy, but the virus itself seems oblivious to this, and spreads worldwide in awesome proportions. Although there are a number of arguments surrounding the ethical and moral aspects of HIV and migration, the situation is complex. One final thought on the issues is this: if we are prepared to say that some citizens from other countries have a right to enter ours because of their special needs, is there any reason to limit the types of need we recognize as relevant? In discussing refugees, for example, we talk in political and sometimes economic terms, but what about health needs? Might it be appropriate to say that, far from being a reason to refuse people entry to a country, a positive HIV status might qualify them for entry on grounds of illnesses which create special needs in the patient which cannot be met in their own country? However, AIDS may be different in that it is a peculiarly social illness, and in some countries it carries with it many of the problems more commonly associated with political persecution or economic deprivation. Furthermore, it is a particular cruelty of the virus that it has struck with so much force in parts of the world economically unable to fight it. Combining these factors there may be room to argue that knowing someone is potentially HIV positive gives us an extra reason to welcome them into our country so that we can share with them some of the resources and knowledge which could benefit them.

In conclusion it is poignant to note that societies sit back, at times helpless, simply observing as the virus hurtles into Asia, entrenches itself across Africa, South America, and proceeds within North America, the Pacific and Europe. Unless policy makers pause and contemplate their policies and their ramifications, they run the risk of losing the battle.

References

ALLEN, D., LEHMAN, S., GREEN, T., LINDEGREN, M., ONORATO, I. and FORRESTER, W. (1994) 'HIV infection among homeless adults and runaway youth United States 1989–92', *AIDS*, **8**, pp. 1593–8.

BARONGO, L., BORGDORFF, W., MOSHA, F., NICOLL, A., GROSSKURTH, H., SENKORO, K., NEWEL, J., CHANGALUCHA, J., KLOKKE, A., KILLEWO, J., VELEMA, J., HAYES, R., DUNN, D., MULLER, L. and RUGEMALILA, J. (1992) 'The epidemiology of HIV-1 infection in urban areas, roadside settlements and rural villages in Mwanza Region, Tanzania', *AIDS*, **6**, pp. 1521–8.

BONNEUX, L., VAN DER STUYFT, P. and TAELMAN, H. (1988) 'Risk factors for infection with HIV among European expatriates in Africa', *British Medical Journal*, **27**, pp. 581–4.

CARSWELL, J., LLOYD, G. and HOWELSS, J. (1989) 'Prevalence of HIV in east-African lorry drivers', *AIDS*, **3**, pp. 759–61.

COHN, S., KLEIN, J., MOHR, J., VAN DER HORST, C.M. and WEBBER, D. (1994) 'The geography of AIDS patterns of urban and rural migration', *Southern Medical Journal*, **87**, 6, pp. 559–606.

COMMUNICABLE DISEASE REPORT (1992) 'AIDS and HIV-1 infection in the UK monthly report', *Communicable Disease Report*, **2**, pp. 137–40.

COWAN, D., BURNDAGE, F. and POMERANTZ, R. (1994) 'The incidence of HIV infection among men in the United States Army Reserve Components 1985–91', *AIDS*, **8**, pp. 505–11.

DECOSAS, J. (1991) 'The demographic AIDS trap for women in Africa: Implications for health promotion', VII Int AIDS Conference, Florence, Italy.

ERIN, C. (1995) Migration Paper Presented at the Prague Meeting of the European AIDS Ethics and Justice group, 1995.

FAIRCHILD, A. and TYNAN, E. (1994) 'Policies of containment immigration in the era of AIDS', *American Journal of Public Health*, **84**, 12, pp. 2011–22.

GARLAND, F., GARLAND, C., GORHAM, E., MILLER, M., CUNNION, S., BERG, S. and BALAZS, L. (1993) 'Lack of association of HIV sero-conversion with visits to foreign prostitutes in US navy personnel', *Archives of Internal Medicine*, **153**, 23, pp. 2685–91.

GILMORE, N., ORKIN, A., DUCKETT, M. and GROVER, S. (1989) 'International travel and AIDS', *AIDS*, **3**, suppl., pp. 225–30.

GOSTIN, L., CLEARY, P., MEYER, K., BRANDT, A. and CHITTENDEN, E. (1990) 'Screening international travellers for the HIV', *New England Journal of Medicine*, **322**, pp. 1743–6.

GUTMAN, L.T. (1994) 'Sexually transmitted disease in children and adolescents with HIV infection', in PIZZO, P. and WILFERT, C. (Eds) *Pediatric AIDS: The Challenge of HIV Infection in Infants, Children and Adolescents*, Baltimore: Williams & Wilkins.

HARRIS, J. (1995) European Ethics Justice and the Law Symposium, Prague.

HAWKES, S., HART, G., JOHNSON, A., SHERGOLD, C., ROSS, E., HERBERT, K., MORTIMER, P., PARRY, J. and MABEY, D. (1994) 'Risk behaviour and HIV prevalence in international travellers', *AIDS*, **8**, pp. 247–52.

HOSHINO, K. (1995) 'HIV/AIDS related bio-ethical issues in Japan', *Bioethics*, **9**, 3/4, pp. 303–8.

HOUWELING, H. and COUTINHO, R. (1991) 'Risk of HIV infection among Dutch expatriates in subSaharan Africa', *International Journal of STDs and AIDS*, **2**, pp. 252–7.

KIRBY, M. (1989) Plenary Address, Montreal International AIDS Conference.

NEWELL, M.L. (1995) Paper presented to the meeting on Caesarean Section and HIV, London.

NOONE, A., GILL, O., CLARKE, S. and PORTER, K. (1991) 'Travel, heterosexual intercourse and HIV-1 infection', *Communicable Dis Rev*, **1**, R, pp. 39–43.

NUNN, A., WAGNER, H., KALAI, A., KENGEYA KAYONDO, J. and MULDER, D. (1995) 'Migration and HIV-1: Sero-prevalence in a rural Ugandan population', *AIDS*, **9**, 5, pp. 503–6.

OPPENHEIM, L.S. (1994) 'Immigration and HIV infection: A pilot study', *AIDS Education and Prevention*, **6**, 1, pp. 74–80.

OVER, M. and PIOT, P. (1992) 'HIV infection and sexually transmitted diseases: The World Bank health sectors priorities review', in JAMISON, D.T. and MOSLEY, W.K.H. (Eds) *Disease Control Priorities in Developing Countries*, New York: Oxford University Press for the World Bank.

PLUMMER, F., MOSES, S. and NDINYA ACHOLA, J. (1991) 'Factors affecting female to male transmission of HIV-1: Implications of transmission dynamics for prevention', in CHEN, L., AMOR, J.S. and SEGAL, S.J. (Eds) *AIDS and Women's Reproductive Health*, New York: Plenum.

QUINN, T. (1994) 'Population migration and the spread of types 1 and 2 HIV', *Proc Natl Acad Sci*, **91**, 7, pp. 2407–14.

RICHARDSON, C., ANCELLE PARK, R. and PAPAEVANGELOU, G. (1993) 'Factors associated with HIV sero-positivity in European injecting drug users', *AIDS*, **7**, 11, pp. 1485–91.

RYDER, R., NDULU, M. and HASSIG, S. (1990) 'Heterosexual transmission of HIV-1 among employees and their spouses at two large businesses in Zaire', *AIDS*, **4**, pp. 725–32.

SANDERS, D. and SAMBO, A. (1991) 'AIDS in Africa: The implication of economic recession and structural adjustment', *Health Policy and Planning*, **6**, pp. 157–65.

SEMPRINI, A., CASTAGNA, C., RAVIZZA, M., FIORE, S., SAVASI, V., MUGGIASCA, M.L., GROSSI, E., GUERRA, B., TIBALDI, C., SCARAVELLI, G., PRATI, E. and PARDI, G. (1995) 'The incidence of complications after Caesarean section in 156 HIV positive women', *AIDS*, **9**, pp. 913–17.

SHERR, L. (1991) *AIDS and HIV Infection in Mothers and Babies*, Oxford: Blackwell Scientific Publications.

SHERR, L. (1993a) 'Ante-natal HIV testing', in SQUIRE, C. (Ed.) *AIDS, Women and Psychology*, London: Sage Publications.

SHERR, L. (1993b) 'Counselling issues for women of reproductive age', in JOHNSON, M. and JOHNSTONE, F. (Eds) *AIDS and Women*, Edinburgh: Churchill Livingstone.

SHERR, L. (1995) 'Psychosocial services of providing care for women with HIV infection' in MINKOFF, H., DeHOVITZ, J. and DUERR, A. (Eds), *HIV Infection in Women*, New York: Raven Press, pp. 107–24.

SHTARKSHALL, R.A. (1995) 'Testing a policy decision: What can happen when you screen for HIV', in FITZSIMONS, D., HARDY, V. and TOLLEY, K. (Eds) *The Economic and Social Impact of AIDS in Europe*, pp. 207–18, London: Cassell.

SINGH, Y. and MALAVIVYA, A. (1994) 'Long-distance truckdrivers in India: HIV infection and their possible role in disseminating HIV into rural areas', *Int J STD AIDS*, **5**, 2, pp. 137–8.

STRICOF, R.L., KENNEDY, J.T., NATTELL, T.C., WEISFUSE, I.B. and NOUICK, L.F. (1991) 'HIV sero-prevalence in a facility for runaway and homeless adolescents', *American Journal of Public Health*, **81**, suppl., pp. 50–3.

VITTECOQ, D., ROUE, R. and MAYAUD, C. (1987) 'AIDS after travelling in Africa: An epidemiological study in seventeen Caucasian patients', *Lancet*, **ii**, pp. 612–14.

WAWER, M., SERWADDA, D., MUSGRAVE, S., KONDELULU, J., MUSAGARA, M. and SEWANKAMBO, N. (1991) 'Dynamics of spread of HIV-1 infection in a rural district in Uganda', *British Medical Journal*, **303**, pp. 1303–6.

WILKINS, A., HAYES, R. and ALONSO, P. (1991) 'Risk factors for HIV-2 infection in the Gambia', *AIDS*, **5**, pp. 1127–32.

YELIBI, S., VALENTI, P., VOLPE, C., CAPRARA, A., DEDY, S. and TAPE, G. (1993) 'Sociocultural aspects of AIDS in an urban peripheral area of Abidjan', *AIDS Care*, **5**, 2, pp. 187–97.

Chapter 6

Migrants and AIDS:
Themes of Vulnerability and Resistance

Renée Sabatier

AIDS has become, to borrow a phrase, an 'incredibly powerful semantic constellation' (Esteva, 1993) whose symbols both record and are used as instruments in continuing struggles between unequally powerful actors. A battleground for different conceptions of morality, representations of AIDS also reflect assumptions concerning disease and illness across diverse cultures. In global discourses on AIDS, biomedical language and assumptions trump those of other actors, privileging clinical definitions of AIDS over other ways of representing the disease. Yet AIDS is clearly as expressive of social and cultural facts as it is of biological ones. Its symptoms and progression can be related to interactions between the individual body, the social body and the body politic, for 'Sickness is not just an isolated event or an unfortunate brush with nature. It is a form of communication — the language of the organs — through which nature, society and culture speak simultaneously (Lock and Scheper-Hughes, 1990, p. 71). Since the language of body organs requires interpretation in order to render it therapeutically intelligible, the question then becomes 'in whose words [will] the body speak?' (Treichler, 1992a, p. 75). The struggle to speak for the bodies of those affected by AIDS defines a 'global culture of AIDS' which, some would argue, implicitly assumes that 'the cultural practices and beliefs of countries are *not all that different*' (Herdt, 1992, p. 8) and, therefore, the AIDS pandemic is amenable to professional management and ultimate control.

An essential tool of professional control is the management of language and meanings — the power to assimilate, coopt or subvert non-medical discourses. This is why, as Kleinman points out, the participation of other disciplines and actors in medicine so often produces not dialogue, but an 'enriched biomedical monologue' (Gaines and Hahn, 1985). Issues of linguistic control are important for all those affected by AIDS, especially for minorities and migrants, whose relative isolation and powerlessness in the larger society is embodied, literally, in specific patterns of illness and disease.

Kleinman (1986) argues that the body mediates social structures and cultural meanings, 'making them part of our physiology' (p. 195). If this is so then we cannot formulate an accurate representation of AIDS without understanding its socio-cultural contexts and the way these are 'read' by the body. Unless migrants and minority communities forge and utilize these readings for themselves, there is danger that 'irreconcilable conflicts of interest . . . will be "negotiated" by those who hold the upper hand, albeit in terms of a language and practice which denies such manipulation and the existence of unequal control' (Taussig, 1980, p. 12). Thus the first principle of AIDS prevention and care for these communities ought to be the promotion of self-organization as an antidote to discrimination and linguistic control, even where social, economic or legal barriers seem to militate against this. The body of the individual vulnerable to or sick with AIDS is no mere medical object but a terrain where 'social truths and special contradictions are played out, as well as a locus of personal and social resistance, creativity and struggle' (Lock and Scheper-Hughes, 1990, p. 71).

This chapter outlines themes relating to the special vulnerabilities of migrants and minorities to HIV and AIDS. It touches first on the social production of AIDS stigma, and then sketches some examples of conditioning factors, deriving from European colonial laws and institutions, which increase migrant risk of HIV infection. The examples used are drawn from interviews conducted with migrants from southern Africa. The chapter briefly touches on the theme of migrant resistance resources as an important consideration in the formulation of prevention and care strategies, and concludes with an argument in support of programmes which promote social learning on AIDS among migrant communities, and which assist the creation and development of peer programmes and community-based organizations.

AIDS and Stigmatization

AIDS appeared in the United States at a time when anxiety reactions to the sexual liberation and homosexual emancipation movements had not yet crystallized, and when the discovery of antibiotics had reduced the terrors of sexually transmitted diseases, particularly syphilis. Gilman argues that this was a time when western culture was left with a potent store of syphilis-related symbols 'but without a sufficiently powerful disease with which to associate these images' (Gilman, 1988, p. 258). AIDS became the object of these anxieties and symbols, absorbing the full weight of historic associations between venereal disease and sin, deviance and social disintegration. From the outset the AIDS epidemic was cast as a cultural war, a battle of meanings and interpretations as much as a war on a virus. A society which feels threatened, Douglas (1966) argues, responds by intensifying the controls which regulate its margins. 'Any structure of ideas is vulnerable at its margins'

(p. 121), and those relegated to the margins are damaged by contact with the danger zone, their social identity marred or polluted. Brandt (1987) summarizes three types of 'spoiled identity' or stigma distinguished in Goffman's (1963, p. 194) classic analysis:

> The first is an abomination of the body; clearly AIDS and all venereal diseases could be so categorised. The second is a blemish of individual character; again victims of sexually transmitted diseases have traditionally been seen as . . . immoral and promiscuous. And third, Goffman identified the tribal stigmas of race, nation or religion . . . the notion that particular groups were especially prone to infection. Perhaps the sexually transmitted diseases carry a particularly weighty stigma because they cut through each of these categories.

The depiction of AIDS as a 'made in the USA' disease of extreme sexual deviance continues to hamper AIDS prevention and advocacy, particularly in societies where traditional beliefs and ways of life are felt to be threatened. Writing on AIDS and stigma, Herek *et al.* (1990) cite comments by Pat Buchanan, an American contender in the 1996 Republican Party presidential primaries: 'There is one, and only one, cause of the AIDS crisis — the wilful refusal of homosexuals to cease indulging in the immoral, unnatural, unsanitary, unhealthy and suicidal practice of anal intercourse, which is the primary means by which the AIDS virus is being spread . . . to others' (p. 120). Widely publicized statements like this by American public figures help to legitimize the stigmatization in other parts of the world of minorities affected by AIDS. An African reprise of Buchanan's words can be heard in a recent denunciation by the Zimbabwean president of homosexuals in his country (*Zimbabwe Herald*, 1995) as 'worse than dogs and pigs' (Drogin, 1995; Jackson, 1995). The president dismissed a letter signed by seventy US congressmen, led by an openly gay house representative, protesting his remarks: 'Let the Americans keep their sodomy, bestiality — stupid and foolish ways' (McNeil, 1995). Most affected by these remarks were young Zimbabwean gays and lesbians, whether living in the country or abroad. For example, Zimbabwean students resident in London have felt repercussions of the president's views, as one of them explains:

> I am afraid to socialise with gay friends or go to gay clubs because I know that some of the other Zimbabwean [students] might see me and report on me to my parents. We are quite a close-knit community in the colleges; everyone knows everyone else and which part of Zimbabwe you come from. Coming to London was the first time I felt I could really be myself without fear. Being able to have gay friends, and having a steady gay partner, has helped me to be more confident and stable. I realise now that at home I was always

somewhat depressed. I felt isolated and so turned to my studies, in which I did well. But there is more to life than studying until you are blind. Now I'm afraid again. I'm afraid to be with one partner so when I'm really lonely I go to clubs and pick up strangers. It's as if all my fears have caught up with me. . . . (Author interview, September 1995)

Migrant stigmatization linked to AIDS began with Haiti, the world's 'first underdeveloped nation' (Farmer, 1992). Why did American epidemiologists speculate that AIDS was brought to the United States by Haitians? Farmer's indispensable ethnography of AIDS in Haiti establishes that this 'parish of the poor' (p. 259), this 'strange and hopelessly diseased country remarkable chiefly for its extreme isolation from the rest of the civilized world' (p. 4), was stigmatized because it was vulnerable, and that 'Haitian origins' theories represent '*a systematic misreading* of the epidemiological and ethnographic data' (p. 2). Misreadings are inevitable, Krieger and Fee (1994) contend, since race and gender classification of health data seems natural to Americans. 'This is how we organise our social life as a nation. To the extent that the presumed biologic categories of race and gender are privileged, exploration of the socio-economic determinants or the historical and cultural contexts of ill health is "suppressed and repressed"' (p. 265). Farmer attrributes the rapid rise of HIV infection in Haiti to economically driven (chiefly male) prostitution, and asks: 'Why might Haiti have been particularly vulnerable to such a commodification of sexuality? In a country as poor as Haiti — "the poorest country in the hemisphere" — AIDS might be thought of as an occupational hazard for workers in the tourist industry' (p. 145). An urban legend recounted in several North American cities sums up the tide of AIDS discrimination against stigmatized expatriate Haitians: 'Almost overnight the Haitian taxi drivers just disappeared. Taxi owners were sure the Haitians would scare away customers, because everyone thought they'd have AIDS. Now the cab drivers in this town are all Pakistani (or Lebanese, Sikh, Iranian, Somali, etc.).'

The linkage between homosexuality, stigma, racism and AIDS, shaped in the American context of the early 1980s, stilll inhibits preventive strategies and the organization of stigmatized communities, whether in Africa or among black communities in the United States (Thomas and Quinn, 1991 and 1993). A history of racist sexually transmitted disease control in African-American communities, particularly the infamous 40-year Tuskegee study (the 'longest non-therapeutic experiment on human beings in medical history', Jones, 1993), makes it difficult for blacks to trust a white AIDS establishment and fuels a fatalism that says 'every bad disease affects us' (Quimby, 1992, p. 163). As Haitian graffiti artists put it: 'AIDS — it had to happen' (Farmer, 1992, p. 259). This sense of the inevitability of AIDS-linked discrimination is echoed by Viviane, a Rwandan commercial sex worker who lived in France until 1989, and who now works in the east-African port of Mombassa part of each year:

I did this work [sex work] in Marseilles for six years. They thought I was beautiful. I had lots of customers, I had money and I lived like a white person. Then they said we African women were spreading AIDS. They called us names in the street and they said we smelled bad. My landlord threw me out of my apartment. The owner of the club where I danced also threw me out. Many of the shopkeepers I knew well refused to serve me. Maybe it was because all of these were among my best customers. So I came home to Africa. I still look good and some of these men search for me each time they are in Mombassa. I will tell you a funny thing. These men are just like the ones I went with in Marseilles. They dress the same, they eat and drink the same, they have the same money and they want the same thing. But here they don't call me 'black pig' and 'dirty monkey' and treat me like I have a disease. We are in Africa now. Here there is no Monsieur Le Pen. Here they don't have to treat me badly just to show their neighbours what good Frenchmen they are. (Author interview, April 1992)

Ten years after the Haitian stigmatization, the US Centers for Disease Control Office of Minority Health produced a workshop report (1993) which overturned the entire presumed basis for racially linked AIDS risk categorization:

Because most associations between diseases and race have no bio-logic basis, race — as a biological concept — 'diverts attention from underlying risk factors' [1993, p. 12]. Further, 'the use of race and ethnicity data in surveillance may reinforce stereotyping, mistrust, and racism ... foster stereotyping and stigmatisation ... [and] an inapropriate 'minority model' of public health and health care, sug-gesting that affected sub-populations are 'high risk', 'hard to reach', 'hard to serve', or 'noncompliant' (p. 13). The final recommenda-tion stated simply that the CDC and other US government agencies should 'Conduct analyses to document the effects of racism (p. 16).

The Construction of Migrant Vulnerability to AIDS

The vulnerability of migrants is closely linked to their relation to power in the host society (Gorovitz, 1994) and the degree of discrimination they experience. Household and community characteristics influence migration, which can be considered an economic or political risk-reduction strategy for many households. Throughout much of the world, residues of colonialism influence the patterning of HIV transmission. The example of the migration history and patterns in southern and east Africa bears on this point. Zimbabwe exemplifies a 'ping pong' epidemiology of HIV between rural and urban areas. Zimbabweans from all socio-economic groups 'retain their links with "home areas" and travel there relatively frequently . . . our labour system would . . . raise the overall rate of spread while simultaneously reducing rural–urban differences' (Davies, 1990, p. 5). Despite one of the best health systems in Africa and a national STD treatment programme, Zimbabwe has been unable to control its high rates of sexually transmitted infection. In the early 1990s close to a million new infections annually were being reported in a population of just over 11 million. Migration-related family separation and men with multiple sexual partners place faithful married women at risk. Such women constitute the majority of women patients at major STD clinics. Simultaneously, a growing number of women are having to become extra-marital partners of men with jobs, simply in order to survive.

Zimbabwe's migrant labour system has its roots in the colonial history of land alienation and restricted urban settlement, managed through a 'uniquely racist ideology' (Moyo, 1995, p. 44). More recently years of drought and the rigours of economic structural adjustment (ESAP), have pushed increasing numbers of people to seek work in the towns. British social engineering of colonial cities was designed to facilitate plentiful supplies of urban male labour while externalizing the maintenance costs of these workers to rural home areas. In Rhodesia in the first half of this century women's legal position was such that 'A single woman is not entitled to municipal housing even if she has children. She is legally a minor, whatever her age, and cannot enter into a contract or lease. There is no question here of the guardian's permission: it is against the present housing policy . . .' (The *Woman's Guide to the Law Through Life,* 1970, quoted in Weiss, 1986, p. 47). Larson (1989) observes that 'Independence has not altered the ambivalence and outright hostility generated towards urban women during the colonial era . . . the sentiment that women did not belong in the cities remained.' However, British colonial officials had no qualms about importing women sex workers to pacify male workers uprooted from their families. Companies in Zimbabwe, for example, brought migrant Zairian women to mining compounds in Huange. British colonial policies in east Africa are thought to have precipitated the migration to Nairobi of tribal Haya women from Bukoba in Tanzania, as well as Ganda women from Uganda, helping to drive women from these tribal groups into prostitution (Southall and Gutkind, 1980).

Supplementary sexual bartering in various forms including commercial sex work can be expedient at some points in the lives of women who increasingly support their households with little or no male participation. An interview with Vesta, a striking and evidently fatigued 26-year old Zimbabwean woman illustrates the point. Vesta partially supports her mother and younger brothers in their rural home while she lives with her children in a small room in Mbare (a high density district in Harare). She was made redundant from her secretarial job due to economic restructuring and now works as a 'bar girl' at night and newspaper vendor during the day:

> I go to the bars, it is true, but I am not a prostitute. I do not live for men's pleasure. Most of the men I go with have been drinking a lot and the thing is really quite easy. It's over in no time. They work hard and are lonely because they are away from home, so they drink. Working in the bars means I can look after my kids during the day, and my sister keeps them at night. If I wasn't working in the bars I would surely be giving carpet interviews, [a form of sexual harassment by prospective employers; the Zimbabwean equivalent of the 'casting couch'] so what is the difference? At home I might have to brew beer, and that is not much better. Why are we women called 'prostitutes' when we come to town looking for work? They say we are responsible for the spread of AIDS, but what about these men? How else am I going to feed my children, which the father fails to support? (Author interview, December 1992)

Writing on prostitution and tourism in south-east Asia, Truong (1990) contextualizes the demographic and labour market changes experienced in many developing countries today. The situation of women becomes one in which 'Traditional reproduction functions connected with the family and kinship system became broken and commoditized along with the commoditization of labour power . . . As new forms of production were introduced, the value of [women's sexuality] changed and their labour became a new form of property, forcing them to use it in the ways which could meet their survival needs under the new conditions' (*ibid.*, p. 76). Truong emphasizes that women's 'reproduction functions have not changed, but only have become disintegrated'.

Joyous, a quick 31-year-old Zimbabwean woman with a dry incessant cough, is one of the growing number of 'new' women migrants. Joyous started selling vegetables when her husband left her. With her profit she bought maize which she paid to have ground and transported to town. She sold the maize meal in small quantities (during the 1992 drought maize was sold by the cupful) in local markets, enabling her to double her funds to purchase *mazitye*, or used clothes, also sold at profit. Now she buses to Johannesburg four times a year where she buys kitchen goods at wholesale prices from Indian shops open twenty-four hours to cater to buyers like her. She is a *mudhira*, a 'dealer'. Her trading activities support four children, her sister's family of five, and at times other relatives. There are occupational hazards in Joyous' work, which involve various sexual pay-offs ('lobbying' is the term often used in Zimbabwe to denote this type of sexual networking) to market officials, immigration police, bus and lorry drivers, merchants, flop-house landlords, and other men encountered along her route.

Like Joyous, Imelda, a 33-year-old Zambian mother of five, makes her living selling. She trades in *saluala,* the used clothing, especially American, which has in recent years become hugely popular (Hansen, 1994, pp. 514–15). She buys 40–50 kilogram bales from large trading firms, and sometimes has to 'lobby' truckers in order to transport the heavy bales. But she sleeps with fewer men now, and can choose them more carefully, than when she formerly worked as a bargirl. Joyous and Imelda are typical of millions of enterprising African women who earn a living in the informal sector, through strategies involving various forms of informal or internal migration, and who are increasingly the major support of their female-headed households. Colonial and gender repression and illegal status too often force their entrepreneurial energy into prostitution. Martha, a 20-year-old market woman in a large Tanzanian town, recounts her experience:

> Selling sardines is a good job, I support my children and the other women are all my friends. But sometimes the market inspector says: 'Where is your licence?' When I show him my licence he says there is something wrong with it, and [that] I will have to pay money to get it stamped. He says I can pay him by sleeping with him. He comes back each day and [harasses] me. I am afraid of his [desire] for my body . . . Finally I sought help from [a community AIDS organization] which took a video of this inspector [harassing] me and the other market women. They showed him the video and told him they will show it in the community if he doesn't leave us alone. They tried to educate him about AIDS. Condoms aren't the only way to fight AIDS! (Author interview, April 1994)

The action of the community AIDS organization mentioned in Martha's story was unconventional but effective. It illustrates the extent to which current male-focused AIDS prevention dogmas and strategies have failed women. Their masculine orientation, preoccupied with condoms and the sex act itself, reinforces women's experiences of alienation not only from their bodies but from the social sources of their power. AIDS prevention strategies neglect the universe of women's relationships — to other women, to their children, their families and communities — which balances, constrains and influences the male–female inequality in power. To conceptualize effective AIDS action for women, it is necessary to eliminate the bias which envisions women as atomistic, male-identified, receptive and dependent beings. Women's own narratives, such as the ones briefly presented here, are often portraits of strength which comes to fruition through relationships and in community. Women participate in a multitude of informal social networks within which they are neither powerless nor victims, but creative actors who mobilize the sometimes meagre resources available to them in surprisingly effective ways.

Resistance Resources, Migration and AIDS

Research on migrants and other diseases suggests that two factors, social networks and support, and personal coping resources, influence the risk of falling ill due to migration stresses. Together these factors comprise a migrant individual or community's resistance resources. Put simply, those with the fewest resistance resources are the most vulnerable to illness (Dressler, 1990, p. 256). Social relationships can contribute to good health in at least three ways: by creating secure zones of social contact and affection; by reducing or mediating interpersonal conflict and tension; and by exerting a buffering effect in times of acute and chronic stress (Williams and House, 1991). In an unequal world, access to social support and the ability to develop successful personal coping skills are linked to one's social position and experiences (Dressler, 1988; Evans *et al.*, 1994). Central to migrant vulnerability to HIV and AIDS are the personal and cultural strengths which they bring on the journey. Pre-migration experiences are known to influence adjustment. For example, Vietnamese immigrants were observed to suffer post-traumatic stress disorder connected with the Vietnam War (August and Gianola, 1987), as do migrants from Rwanda and the former Yugoslavia. Mexican women migrating to the United States were better adjusted when they had stronger pre-migration support and could maintain contact with their pre-migration support network (Vega *et al.*, 1987). The literature on illness and resistance resources is complex and there is inadequate space here to explore its relevance for AIDS prevention and care. However, two contrasting examples of community responses to AIDS suggest a number of themes and issues worth exploring in relation to migration and AIDS.

Puerto Rican migrants to the United States run an extremely high risk of acquiring HIV (Selik *et al.*, 1992). A commonwealth of the United States, Puerto Rico faces 'special obstacles in its efforts to combat [HIV] ... commonwealth status has created ambiguity in the relationship [with] the federal government ... there are inconsistencies regarding the island's participation in federal studies of health status, and in how much funding is made available to the island for federal health programs' (Bermudez and Diaz, 1993, p. 5). Large-scale economic migration to the United States began in the late 1940s, paralleled by a sharp rise in intravenous use, particularly in black and Puerto Rican ghettos in northern (US) cities. The extreme fluidity of the migration pattern between Puerto Rico and the United States makes it difficult to determine the actual numbers of individuals going back and forth (Perez, 1993). Puerto Rican men have the lowest labour force participation rates of any ethnic or racial group in the US. By 1990, AIDS was the leading cause of death for Puerto Rican men and women between twenty-five and forty-four years, much higher than for Latino men and women as a whole. Puerto Ricans have the largest number of AIDS cases of any Spanish-speaking subgroup in the US (Selik *et al.*). One reason for the higher prevalence of HIV infection due to injecting drug use among Puerto Ricans is that 'sterile needles may be more available to whites, and whites may be more able to afford them' (Rogers and Walter, 1987). Another reason may be that Puerto Ricans are a widely stigmatized ethnic group in the United States. They sometimes seem to be too American for other Latinos and too Latino for other Americans. Their low status and conflicted identity influence both individual self-esteem and the ability of their communities to secure resources to cope with AIDS. In consequence their resistance to the AIDS epidemic has yet to be articulated in the organizational forms which could promote shared learning and augment coping behaviours.

Uganda offers a contrasting example. Though it has suffered a devastating level of HIV infection, much of it contracted before AIDS was named, Uganda has rallied to combat the disease and finally appears to be having some success in levelling the incidence of new infections. Ugandan society reached a nadir just before the advent of AIDS during years of civil strife and war associated with ousting the dictatorships of Idi Amin and Milton Obote. The country's infrastructure was destroyed, its social relationships undermined and its political institutions fragmented and perverted. Out of these ruins rose a strong desire to rebuild as a nation, and a desire to bear witness, to speak the truth about the horrors of the civil conflict. Uganda's president, Yoweri Museveni, spoke publicly about AIDS long before most other African and world leaders. The pragmatic and non-stigmatizing approach adopted was summarized by the head of the National AIDS Programme in 1987: 'There is a snake in the house. Do you just sit there and ask where the snake came from?' (Sabatier, 1988, p. 148). Uganda produced the first African AIDS service organization. In 1986, Noerine Kaleeba, a Ugandan whose husband was studying in the UK, learned that he had AIDS, a disease they had never heard of. On her husband's death she and fifteen others, twelve of whom had AIDS, founded TASO, a Kampala-based AIDS counselling and peer support organization. As Kaleeba explains: 'When we began we were just a group of lunatic people, some of whom had AIDS. We met to talk, to cry, to pray, to share, to let off steam. Soon we realized we needed to do more than that' (Kaleeba *et al.*, 1991, p. 49). TASO pioneered AIDS counselling in Africa, putting its own distinctive stamp on the therapeutic situation. The organization attempted to cover the whole country by starting and supporting local branches. Using a peer-based model, TASO counsels tens of thousands of AIDS-affected Ugandans each year, and trains hundreds of AIDS counsellors. Because it exists Uganda has one of, if not the, best AIDS counselling programmes in Africa. The spirit in which Noerine Kaleeba could found TASO also led the pop musician, Philly Lutaaya, to go public with the illness in his music and in a film called 'Born in Africa'. Thus through the actions of courageous individuals, and because post-civil war Ugandans were used to organizing survival at community level, the fear and victimization surrounding AIDS was gradually overcome.

What resistance resources did Uganda bring to the struggle against AIDS?

Kleinman (1986, p. 168) states that 'The social sources of human distress are local human contexts that distribute resources unequally, that transmit the effects of large-scale socio-political, economic, and ecological forces unjustly, and that place particular categories of persons under greatest social pressure.' Uganda is not dominated economically or culturally by its former colonial power. The country and its president have laid enormous stress on the need to pull together in order to recover from the war years. Materially disadvantaged in comparison with Puerto Ricans, Ugandans have achieved high educational levels relative to other African countries. By contrast Puerto Rico is still a *de facto* colony of the United States and is both overshadowed and under-financed by its huge neighbour. A chief source of income is American tourism, including sex tourism. Puerto Rican educational attainment and per capita income is extremely low relative to that of other Americans. To a far greater extent than Ugandans, Puerto Ricans are exposed to the aspirations of western mass culture without the resources to realize them. Most importantly, the Puerto Rican AIDS epidemic is related to the use of prohibited injectable drugs, so that organizing around AIDS runs into all the dilemmas involved in organizing any 'illegal' group. The combination of community and individual resources and skills on which Ugandans were able to draw has been unavailable in the Puerto Rican situation. It is no coincidence that the two countries of the western hemisphere most affected by HIV and AIDS are Haiti and Puerto Rico — both peripheralized client states of their vastly more powerful American neighbour.

Conclusion

The argument advanced in this chapter is that it is not possible to formulate an adequate understanding of migrant needs and exposure to HIV without attending to the ways in which the migrants themselves experience and represent their condition. This is especially true for informal, irregular and clandestine migrants, who fear the interest of strangers, however well-intentioned. As Ignatieff (1986) has written 'There are few presumptions in human relations more dangerous than the idea that one knows what another human being needs better than they do themselves' (p. 11). Understanding migrant experiences requires specific knowledge of their local contexts, the 'nested hierarchies of family, network, work, and community settings' (Kleinman, 1986, p. 168) which influence their choices, risks, vulnerabilities and resistance. AIDS information, seen to be the foremost tool of prevention and care programmes, is always reciprocal; when we emphasize informing vulnerable individuals and communities at the expense of being informed by them, we risk throwing away valuable keys to understanding. Treichler's perceptive formulation is most helpful here:

To believe that information and communication about AIDS will separate fact from fiction and reality from metaphor is to suppress the linguistic complexity of everyday life. Further, to inform is also to perform; to communicate is also to construct and interpret. Information does not simply exist; it issues from and in turn sustains a way of looking at and behaving toward the world; it shapes programmatic agendas and even guides capital investments. (Treichler, 1992b, p. 401)

In the European context Rosenbrock (1993, p. 7) advocates a 'social learning strategy', the 'learning process by which individuals and society can adapt (with a maximum of prevention) to life with HIV'. A recent four-country analysis of AIDS policies and their effects (Steffen, 1994) provides some general lessons. Steffen argues that responses to AIDS in Germany and the UK were more effective than those in France and Italy because, among other factors, homosexual men were politically well-organized and had pre-existing health-focused organizations, and because there was a strong public health tradition. Both of these factors are related to traditions of effective local government and political participation acting in a sphere of autonomy. Italy failed in implementing its national AIDS programme, which was professionalized and non-participatory, but succeeded in legitimizing sexuality and marginal behaviour as public health responsibilities. France had all possible disadvantages, including archaic legislation, over-centralization, and relatively weak non-governmental organizations, including those of gay men. AIDS prevention and care are most effective when the vulnerable speak with their own voice and are able to form service and advocacy organizations in their own communities.

The Global AIDS Policy Coalition comes close to a 'social learning' viewpoint when it says that 'the HIV pandemic flourishes where individuals' capacity to learn and to respond is constrained. Belonging to a discriminated group reduces personal capacity to respond. The practical implication is that interventions are needed to reduce the societal risk factor of discrimination, in order to strengthen the personal capacity of people who are most vulnerable to HIV/AIDS' (GAPC, 1993, p. 7; see also Cook, 1994; and AIDS, Health and Human Rights, 1995). If there exist 'societal risk factors' then there must also exist societal immunity: a degree of protection from risk exposure conferred through membership in a community where learning resources and experiences are shared, elaborated and reproduced. That social immunity can be at least partially restored through community action and the building of coalitions and movements has been demonstrated by the success in reducing HIV transmission among many gay communities and some others such as Australian sex workers and injecting drug users in The Netherlands.

Migrants and minority communities, however, frequently suffer from varying degrees of disruption of social learning (for example see Goicoechea-Balboa, 1994; and Migrant Health Services, 1990). Public health strategies to assist migrant communities to respond to HIV should help to analyse and as much as possible to remove or reduce impediments to social learning (not the same thing as supplying 'AIDS education'). Peer approaches and self-organizations can be an antidote to stigma, recuperating 'spoiled identity'. Pooled resistance resources create and enhance social immunity. There are many sources of the condition of vulnerability to AIDS, and therefore combating it requires a marriage of many strategies, all founded in a practical understanding of the need for recognition and advocacy of migrants' human and legal rights. The integration of care and support with prevention is a helpful measure, since care and support programmes are often an effective entry point into marginalized or clandestine communities. Frequently a critical need among migrants is for advocacy and legal services; in many cases these should take priority over medical approaches, with the latter integrated into the framework of the former, rather than the reverse. Reading the words of a migrant woman with HIV (Chipo, a 39-year-old Zimbabwean), we can identify multiple points at which appropriate support or intervention, not limited to AIDS education or STD treatment, may have prevented her infection:

> What I have learned about this disease . . . is that AIDS is no one thing. AIDS is there when your husband drinks and comes home late at night and beats you and tells you to cook *sadza* [maize meal porridge]. AIDS is there when he loses his job and turns to other women. AIDS is there when the rains don't come and the borehole dries up so you have no water for your children to drink. Then AIDS follows you to town where you are working very hard selling vegetables until the police come and push you out and take away your vegetables and you have no money to buy more. AIDS is when your children are hungry and there is no food because you are being adjusted [referring to structural adjustment policies], so you have to go to the bars. AIDS is there when you baby is sick and the clinic says nothing can be done. Your husband pushes you out of the house and you have not even clothes enough to cover you, so what can you do? He doesn't want to talk about AIDS. Now he is dead. His family comes to take away all the things in the house, so you have nothing. No one is there to help you. It is a long story. That is the story of AIDS. (Author interview, February 1995).

But Chipo did find help at an AIDS support organization and, when she became quite ill and returned to her rural home area, she decided to start another support group there. With the help of a mission hospital she succeeded in bringing together about thirty widows and women with AIDS, and they have started a small tailoring business. Despite her weakening condition Chipo works several hours a day in AIDS counselling and home visits. When shown the above quote several months after it was spoken she commented:

AIDS has opened my eyes. Though my body is weak now, my spirit is strong. It is the spirit of many people fighting AIDS together. I will leave this spirit to my children, and they will have a better life than me. I will die knowing that I have made something important with my life. (Author interview, December 1995)

References

AIDS, HEALTH and HUMAN RIGHTS (1995) International Federation of Red Cross and Red Crescent Societies and the François-Xavier Bagnoud Center for Health and Human Rights, Harvard School of Public Health, Geneva and Cambridge, MA.

AUGUST, L.R. and GIANOLA, B.A. (1987) 'Symptoms of war trauma induced psychiatric disorders: Southeast Asian refugees and Vietnam veterans', *International Migration Review*, **21**, pp. 820–31.

BERMUDEZ, G.M. and DIAZ, J.A. (1993) *HIV/AIDS among Puerto Ricans*, Washington, DC: Center for Health Promotion, National Council of La Raza, November Fact Sheet.

BRANDT, A. (1987) *No Magic Bullet: A Social History of Venereal Disease in the United States Since 1880*, (expanded edition), New York: Oxford University Press.

CENTERS FOR DISEASE CONTROL (1993) 'The use of race and ethnicity in public health surveillance', Summary of the CDC/ARSDR Workshop, *MMWR*, **42** (RR-10), pp. 1–17.

COOK, R.J. (1994) *Women's Health and Human Rights*, Geneva: World Health Organisation.

DAVIES, R. (1990) 'The political economy of AIDS in Zimbabwe', paper presented to the conference on 'The Socio-economic Impact of AIDS', Harare, 14 March.

DOUGLAS, M. (1966) *Purity and Danger: An Analysis of the Concepts of Pollution and Taboo*, London: Routledge & Kegan Paul.

DRESSLER, W.W. (1988) 'Social consistency and psychological distress', *Journal of Health and Social Behaviour*, **29**, pp. 79–91.

DRESSLER, W.W. (1990) 'Culture, stress and disease', in JOHNSON, T.M. and SARGENT, C.F. (Eds) *Medical Anthropology: Contemporary Theory and Method*, New York: Praeger.

DROGIN, B. (1995) 'Mugabe launches an anti-gay crusade', *Montréal Gazette*, 28 August, B1.

ESTEVA, G. (1993) 'Development', in SACHS, G. (Ed.) *The Development Dictionary*, Johannesburg: Witwatersrand University Press.

EVANS, R.G., BARER, M.L. and MARMOR, T.R. (1994) *Why Are Some People Healthy and Others Not?: The Determinants of Health of Populations*, New York: Aldine De Gruyter.

FARMER, P. (1992) *AIDS and Accusation: Haiti and the Geography of Blame*, Berkeley: University of California Press.

GAINES, A.D. and HAHN, R. (Eds) (1985) *Physicians of Western Medicine: Anthropological Approaches to Theory and Practice*, Dordecht, The Netherlands: D. Reidel.

Renée Sabatier

GILMAN, S. (1988) *Disease and Representation*, Ithaca, NY: Cornell University Press.
GLOBAL AIDS POLICY COALITION (1993) *Towards a New Health Strategy for AIDS*, Cambridge, Massachusetts: Harvard School of Public Health.
GOFFMAN, E. (1963) *Stigma: Notes on the Management of Spoiled Identity*, Englewood Cliffs, New Jersey.
GOICOECHEA-BALBOA, A. (1994) 'Why we are losing the AIDS battle in rural migrant communities', *AIDS and Public Policy Journal*, Spring, pp. 36–48.
GOROVITZ, S. (1994) 'Reflections on the Vulnerable', in BANKOWSKI, Z. and BRYANT, J.H. (Eds) *Poverty, Vulnerability, and the Value of Human Life: A Global Agenda for Bioethics*, Geneva: Council for International Organizations of Medical Sciences.
HANSEN, K.T. (1994) 'Dealing with used clothing: *Saluala* and the construction of identity in Zambia's third republic', *Public Culture*, 6, 3, pp. 503–23.
HERDT, G. (1992) 'Introduction', in HERDT, G. and LINDENBAUM, S. (Eds) *The Time of AIDS: Social Analysis, Theory and Method*, Newbury Park, California: Sage.
HEREK, G.M. *et al.* (1990) *Psychological Aspects of Serious Illness: Chronic Conditions, Fatal Diseases, and Clinical Care*, Washington, DC: American Psychological Association.
IGNATIEFF, M. (1986) *The Needs of Strangers: An Essay on Privacy, Solidarity, and the Politics of Being Human*, Harmondsworth, UK: Penguin Books.
JACKSON, D.Z. (1995) 'Mugabe's anti-gay tirade', *Globe and Mail*, 14 August.
JONES, J. (1993) *Bad Blood: The Tuskegee Syphilis Experiment*, (New and expanded edition), New York: The Free Press.
KALEEBA, N., RAY, S. and WILLMORE, B. (1991) *We Miss You All*, Harare, Zimbabwe: Women and AIDS Support Network.
KLEINMAN, A. (1985) 'Introduction', in GAINES, A.D. and HAHN, R. (Eds) *Physicians of Western Medicine: Anthropological Approaches to Theory and Practice*, Dordrecht, The Netherlands: D. Reidel.
KLEINMAN, A. (1986) *Social Origins of Disease and Distress: Depression, Neurasthenia and Pain in Modern China*, New Haven, CT: Yale University Press.
KRIEGER, N. and FEE, E. (1994) 'Man–made medicine and women's health: the biopolitics of sex/gender and race/ethnicity', *International Journal of Health Services*, 24, 2, pp. 265–83.
LARSON, A. (1989) 'The social context of HIV in Africa: Historical and cultural bases of east and central African sexual behaviour', *Review of Infectious Diseases*, 11, pp. 716–31.
LOCK, M. and SCHEPER-HUGHES, N. (1990) 'A critical interpretive approach in medical anthropology: Rituals and routines of discipline and dissent', in JOHNSON, T.M. and SARGENT, C.F. (Eds) *Medical Anthropology: Contemporary Theory and Method*, New York and Westport, CT: Praeger.
McNEIL, D. (1995) 'Gay-bashing thrives at highest political levels but hasn't reached the streets', *Globe and Mail*, 11 September.
MIGRANT HEALTH SERVICES (1990) *Outreach Services to Migrants: The Reality, the Dream*, Rockville, Maryland: US Department of Health and Human Services.
MOYO, S. (1995) *The Land Question in Zimbabwe*, Harare, Zimbabwe: SAPES Books.
PEREZ, S. (1993) *Moving from the Margins: Puerto Rican Young Men and Family Poverty*, Washington, DC: National Council of La Raza, August.

QUIMBY, E. (1992) 'Anthropological witnessing for African Americans: Power, responsibility and choice in the age of AIDS', in HERDT, G. and LINDENBAUM, S. (Eds) *The Time of AIDS: Social Analysis, Theory and Method*, Newbury Park, California: Sage.

ROGERS, M. and WALTER, W. (1987) 'AIDS in Blacks and Hispanics: Implications for prevention', *Issues in Science and Technology*, **3**, pp. 9–96.

ROSENBROCK, R (1993) 'AIDS: Questions and lessons for public health', *AIDS and Public Policy Journal*, **8**, 1, pp. 5–19.

SABATIER, R. (1988) *Blaming Others: Prejudice, Race and Worldwide AIDS*, Philadelphia: New Society Publishers.

SELIK, R.M., CASTRO, K.G. and PAPPAIOANOU, M. (1992) 'Racial/ethnic differences in the risk of AIDS in the United States', quoted in 'The HIV/AIDS epidemic in Puerto Rico' in the *Report of the National Commission on AIDS*, Washington, DC, June.

SOUTHALL, A.W. and GUTKIND, P.C.W. (1980) 'Marriage', in MUGA, E. (Ed.) *Studies in Prostitution: East, West and South Africa, Zaire and Nevada*, Nairobi: Kenya Literature Bureau.

STEFFEN, M. (1994) 'Public policies against AIDS in four western European countries: France, the UK, Italy and Germany', *Current AIDS Literature*, **7**, 10, pp. 352–8.

TAUSSIG, M.T. (1980) 'Reification and the consciousness of the patient', *Social Science and Medicine*, **14B**, pp. 3–13.

THOMAS, S.B. and QUINN, S.C. (1991) 'The Tuskegee Syphilis Study, 1932 to 1972: Implications for HIV education and AIDS risk education programs in the black community', *American Journal of Public Health*, **81**, 11, pp. 1498–505.

THOMAS, S.B. and QUINN, S.C. (1993) 'The burdens of race and history on black Americans' attitudes toward needle exchange policy to prevent HIV disease', *Journal of Public Health Policy*, **14**, 3, pp. 320–47.

TREICHLER, P. (1992a) 'The cultural construction of reality', in HERDT, G. and LINDENBAUM, S. (Eds) *The Time of AIDS: Social Analysis, Theory and Method*, London: Sage.

TREICHLER, P. (1992b) 'AIDS and HIV infection in the Third World: A First World chronicle', in FEE, E. and FOX, D.M. (Eds) (1992) *AIDS: The Making of a Chronic Disease*, Berkeley: University of California Press.

TRUONG, T.-D., (1990) *Sex, Money and Morality: Prostitution and Morality in South-east Asia*, London: Zed Books.

VEGA, W.A., KOLODY, B. and VALLE, J.R. (1987) 'Migration and mental health: An empirical test of depression risk factors among immigrant Mexican women', *International Migrant Review*, **21**, pp. 512–30.

WEISS, R. (1986) *The Women of Zimbabwe*, Harare: Nehanda Publishers.

WILLIAMS, D.R. and HOUSE, J.S. (1991) 'Stress, social support, control and coping: A social epidemiological view', in BADURA, B. and KICKBUSCH, I. (Eds) *Health Promotion Research: Towards a New Social Epidemiology*, Geneva: World Health Organization.

ZIMBABWE HERALD, 2 August 1995.

Chapter 7

Stigma and Racism as they Affect Minority Ethnic Communities

Oonagh O'Brien and Shivananda Khan

It is only natural that they insist on measuring us with the yardstick that they use for themselves forgetting that the ravages of time are not the same for all, and that the quest of our identity is just as arduous and bloody for us as it was for them. The interpretation of our reality through patterns not our own serves only to make us ever more unknown, ever less free, ever more solitary. (Gabriel Garcia Marquez)

People who are directly affected by HIV/AIDS and who are also from ethnic minority groups experience many different levels of racism and stigma, both covert and overt. Although it is always difficult to measure racism, it can be even more difficult to disentangle the multiple experiences of stigma and prejudice when these are compounded by HIV. This chapter examines such experience in two specific minority ethnic groups living in the same place: the United Kingdom. People belonging to one group, the Irish, are largely white, and have full legal rights to travel and work in Britain. The other group, south Asian, are largely black, and are highly restricted in their rights to travel to Britain, although once admitted as legal residents they have the same full rights. The two groups share a history of British colonial rule in the country of origin, of violent conflict to end that rule, and of varied experience of racism and prejudice. Both would identify with Franz Fanon concerning the experience of colonialism:

The colonial migrant in the 'mother' country cannot win. At best s/he can only resist the worst effects of the institutionalised historical relationship between the two cultures. Attempts at assimilation are rebuffed or treated with a certain specific kind of contempt. Attempts to preserve the native culture intact are regarded as open acts of defiance and a denigration of the host culture. Every instance of contact with the colonist Other is potentially fraught with anxiety for the migrant. To be accepted s/he must act in accordance with the stereotypes the host culture imposes as long as they are positive ones of the happy go lucky, easy-going and cheerful native. (Fanon, 1970, quoted in Greenslade, 1991, p. 16)

Both of the ethnic groups described in this chapter have a specific experience of racism and prejudice. Taking on board the issues of AIDS appears to many members of these two groups to be asking for trouble; it is to invite further prejudice and exclusion from the mainstream society in which they are living. Additionally, a central part of the identity of these two groups is linked to a strong ethical and moral code, and closely associated with traditional family structures and religion. To fully understand the impact of the stigma of AIDS on these two ethnic minority groups, it is important to give a brief description of the specific experience of racism and prejudice within each, in its own terms. We will then go on to examine policy implications for the work of community-based organizations working with HIV/AIDS in the two communities. Later, work around prevention care and support will be discussed, with reference to the way in which racism and stigma hinders that work. Lastly, we present future options for models of good practice, and the need for cooperation through networking at European and international levels.

Racism and Prejudice

The word racism refers to negative discrimination on the basis of the physical characteristics and/or the religion or culture of an individual or a group. Racial prejudice can be defined as discrimination based on these same criteria, but without the personal or institutional power to back it up. Although the belief that the world is neatly divided up into different races has long been considered simplistic, we are left with the implications of this belief in the concept of racism. In Britain these shades of meaning have constantly to be renegotiated by minority ethnic groups fighting racism and prejudice.

The Irish Experience in Britain: Oonagh O'Brien

There has been discussion among Irish, and other minority ethnic groups, as to whether a largely white minority ethnic group could be considered to experience racism. Much of this discussion has been influenced by the language of the Race Relations Act passed by the UK Parliament in 1976. This Act, passed as migration from ex-colonies (excluding Ireland) was being severely curtailed, attempted to offer a level of protection to people subject to overtly racist behaviour. The act defines a 'racial group' as a group of persons defined by any reference to 'colour, race, nationality or ethnic or national origins, and references to a person's racial group refer to any racial group into which he [*sic*] falls' (Race Relations Act 1976). That the Irish come within the terms of the Race Relations Act as a distinct racial group has been successfully tested by Irish people taking cases under the terms of the Act (e.g. Haringey Publications, 1991, p. 7).

The daily experience of racism and prejudice by white Irish people in Britain differs in substantial ways from that of black minority ethnic groups. A largely white minority group is a less visible target for racist behaviour. But it has been that very invisibility which has made it difficult for the Irish to collectivize their experiences of racism and prejudice, and to unite as a minority ethnic group to challenge discriminatory behaviour. HIV brings these issues into sharp focus: our argument in this chapter is that a community organization catering to the needs of Irish people affected by HIV/AIDS in Britain, necessarily deals constantly with issues of racism and stigma related both to HIV *and* to ethnic identity.

Hickman and Walter (1995, p. 5) have written: 'The Irish are largely invisible as an ethnic group in Britain, but continue to be racialised as inferior and alien Others.' Hickman (1995) also demonstrates that it is invisibility which has contributed to the racism and stigma Irish people experience in Britain, and argues that the state education system played a role in this by ensuring the separate education of Irish children in Catholic schools, causing further separation from the indigenous population and cloaking ethnic identity in a religious mask. Anti-Irish prejudice took the form of segregation, which further added to invisibility. This invisibility is compounded for Irish women, who, while outnumbering Irish men, are not part of the imagery of the Irish held by the host population. Hickman argues that it is the assumption of the existence of a homogenous 'white' race which has contributed to the invisibility of the Irish: 'It is all too easy for "whiteness" to be equated with an homogeneous way of life. What is necessary is research on the deconstruction of "whiteness"' (Hickman and Walter, 1995, p. 8; see also Allen, 1994, on the importance of re-examining the concept of 'white' as homogenous and unproblematic).

It is estimated that between Irish-born (830 453 in the 1991 census) and second generation, there are up to 2 million Irish people in Britain. The long years of colonization by the British have had a lasting impact on Ireland. The language, the legal system and many other institutions are legacies of British rule. The most evident and widely resented experience of direct discrimination has been through the Prevention of Terrorism Act (PTA) 1974. Under this Act, the British judicial system has wide-ranging powers to detain any Irish person without access to legal advice, or the right to contact their family or friends, for up to seventy-two hours. Up to 86 000 predominately Irish people have been detained for up to an hour under the Act every year between 1987 and 1990 (PTA Research and Welfare Association, 1995). The Act had the effect of spreading a climate of fear, which can be clearly linked to the length of time it has taken for the Irish to organize as a minority ethnic group in Britain.

Despite geographical proximity, and the full legal rights Irish people have to residency and work, the migration process is not an easy one. The data available about Irish people's experiences in Britain reveal a story of discrimination: Irish people experience significant problems in the area of housing, and there is evidence they constitute the largest single ethnic group among the homeless (see O'Meachair *et al.*, 1988; O'Flynn, 1991). Many are employed in unskilled labouring jobs such as building and road making, and in industries with high rates of accidents and deaths, and very little security. Research has demonstrated that, unlike among other ethnic groups, there is a marked deterioration in the health of Irish migrants after migrating to Britain, which can also be seen by the marked increase in Standard Mortality Ratios among Irish people on migration. This increase is even greater in second generation Irish migrants (Raftery *et al.*, 1990; Greenslade, 1991). Irish people have the reputation of only going to health services when they are in a crisis, and extremely ill. Going to the doctor is perceived as a weakness (see Helman, 1990; O'Brien, 1993).

The Irish also make important contributions to the British labour market, however, working in health and social services, the media and business. Theirs is a community whose talents and skills make a rich contribution to British society. Traditionally, services for Irish people in need have been developed through the community itself. These have centred around the Catholic Church and the Irish centres found in most large towns in Britain. As well as being a focus for cultural activities, these centres provide a range of social services. It is important to point out here that, as with any migrant and minority ethnic group, the Irish community is a heterogeneous one. Some Irish people choose to have no contact whatsoever with things Irish once they have migrated: for many of those who chose to organize outside of them, the existing Irish community organizations represent the very values they left Ireland to get away from. This has, at various times particularly applied to gay men, lesbians, single parents, unmarried couples, single women, feminists, and many young people.

It is thus important not to assume that all Irish people affected by HIV/AIDS share the same homogenous culture. For the people to whom these identities can apply, there may be a sense of double marginalization — from mainstream British culture because of being Irish, and from the traditionally conservative Irish community in Britain. This can result in a conflict of identities. As one writer has put it: '. . . it's a bitter option to choose between living [in England] in an anti-Irish culture although surviving as a lesbian, and coming home to face the reactions of friends and family when they discover the "awful truth"' (*Irish Feminist Review*, 1984, p. 143).

The invisibility of the Irish extends to the world of HIV/AIDS. The epidemiology of HIV/AIDS in Ireland is different to that of England.[1,2] In Ireland the major route of transmission has been through injecting drug use, and this is the transmission route given by over half the people with a known HIV diagnosis. In England the overwhelming majority of people known to be HIV positive attribute their infection to sex between men. However, as there is no category for 'Irish' in monitoring of HIV infections in England, the different pattern of epidemiology remains hidden. Services in England, largely geared towards English gay men, are not necessarily appropriate either for the majority of Irish people who are HIV positive or for the special needs of seropositive Irish gay men. This invisibility, combined with the subtle effects of living in an anti-Irish culture, is given as justification for not responding to the needs of Irish people living with HIV. The result is that it is extremely difficult for them to gain access to appropriate services without the support and advocacy of a community-based group. At the same time, while the case for targeted services for black minority ethnic groups is generally accepted, the case for a white one is not, despite extensive evidence of need (O'Brien, 1993; Riordan, 1994).

The exclusion from the Irish community, and the double marginalization Irish people experience living in an anti-Irish culture in Britain, can result in an overwhelming isolation for those diagnosed HIV positive. There is literally no one to turn to; people at home cannot be told of the diagnosis because of the implications that go along with it, yet support ultimately comes from family and communities that are familiar and belong to 'home'.

The South Asian Experience: Shivananda Khan

The south Asian communities reflect a diversity of different languages, cultural frameworks and religious beliefs. There are also differences between urban and rural origins, in whether people come from the Indian subcontinent, east Africa, or the West Indies. Further, there are issues around caste, socio-economic status, and particular religious 'beliefs'. Beyond these differences are the range of specific behaviours, such as those of gay-identified men, men who have sex with men, women who have sex with women, drug users, and sex workers, both female or male. Individual identities may include a strong religious component or not, public beliefs and private perceptions and practice, female value systems, male value systems. South Asians include young people (a group itself not homogenous), unemployed or employed, those who identify as 'black', those who identify themselves as British/English, those who identify with their specific community, (i.e. Asian or Bangladeshi, Pakistani, Gujerati, Punjabi, Tamil, Singhalese, Muslim, Hindu, Buddhist), those who are new immigrants, refugees, old immigrants, first, second, third generation.

We have been defined as black, or as ethnic minority, or minority ethnic, or coloured. We are the Other, arising from different cultures, with different religions and languages and social practices than those from the host culture. We may often wear different clothes, eat different foods, relate to each other in different ways, but most importantly, we are often a different colour. From pale cream to black, we stand visible in the midst of the dominant 'white' European culture, a presence, a demand of visibility to be recognized. The return on this demand incurred by our visibility has been that of *integration*. Our differences must be reduced, but at the same time imperial and colonial history has exoticized and eroticized, demonized and victimized us. So to paraphrase a prominent politician, if we don't support the English cricket team, then we are not British.

In the development of an identity, part of the process is to create the Other, that who cannot share attributes of that identity, and is defined by exclusion. In this development, the framework of prejudice arises. We do not like certain things, attributes, qualities, that the Other apparently possesses by definition. We are prejudiced against them. When the Other is from a different country, or of a different colour, or culture, then this prejudice develops as 'racial' prejudice. We all have to a greater or lesser extent aspects of 'racial prejudice'.

Within European languages, the term 'white' carries hidden assumptions of purity, God, cleanliness, virginity, superiority, life, day time, malehood. The word 'black' carries connections with terms such as evil, Satan, dirty, licentious, unclean, death, women. Non-Europeans have been to a large extent identified with the word 'black' with all the hidden linguistic assumptions. Racial prejudice is not an intellectual exercise. It requires constant vigilance in how we think, what we feel, what we say, how we do things. These connections of language, imagery, perceptions, world views, feelings and emotional responses, reflect the social and cultural perceptions into which a person is born. They are the undercurrents, the invisible assumptions, of the individual or the society's world-view, from which actions and judgements are made.

Over the last four hundred years, European nations had been involved in imperial and colonial subjugation of vast territories of the world. Begun as part of trade with other countries, this rapidly grew into social, political and economic control over different nationalities and cultures. The slave trade and the economic destruction of Moghul India enabled Britain, for example, rapidly to become the leading economic, political and military power. All this needed justification, and out of this search for justification arose the assumption that the British 'race', the 'white race', were morally, culturally and socially superior to any other. Language, the Christian Church, art, literature and other social forms manifested these beliefs and enabled

Europe to carry out its programme of imperialism and colonialism. Racial prejudice became imbued with personal, social and political power to control and construct the Other. Racial prejudice developed into racism. *It is the institutional power dynamics linked with racial prejudice that form racism.* Yet institutions are not abstract phenomena, separate from the people who work in them, who manage them and who create them. Racism, and the power to make it manifest, are part of institutions and their frameworks.

Britain has had a Race Relations Act since 1976, which legally requires people not to practise racial discrimination, but the actual daily practice is shrouded in different perceptions of what this means. We can claim, for instance, that we are delivering services to all people irrespective of their colour, but if these services are so shaped that it becomes difficult for people to gain access to them because of language, social relationships, environment, etc., then, while we may believe we are not racially discriminating, in practice we will be. Those who are part of the institution and part of the host culture have the power to exercise that discrimination and, most importantly, to define it as discriminatory.

This has often led to a denial of cultural diversity and differences between the various communities. A homogenous response is asked for. The 'Other' becomes solidified as an 'ethnic minority'. Community and cultural diversity is reduced to some imagined singular conformity. The result is that, within attempts to address the issues of racism in service delivery, the marginalization of several communities is increased because differences are ignored. Thus, the following scenario can all too often occur: a local health authority, in its efforts to develop more accessible services, employed a 'black' community worker to address the needs of the 'black community'. Unfortunately, the person employed was of Ugandan origin who was supposed to work with a Bangladeshi community! Racism is not only about abusing 'black' people by calling them 'nigger' or 'paki', or by trying to burn their homes, or even killing them. It is also about the day-to-day reality of being constantly defined as less worthy and less able than those of the host culture.

Implications of Racism for HIV/AIDS Service Delivery

Fifteen years on, and with HIV/AIDS having become pandemic in Africa and south Asia, we still hear comments in minority ethnic communities such as, 'it's a white man's disease', 'it's nothing to do with us', 'we are safe because we do not have premarital sex', 'our culture will protect us' or 'there are no homosexuals in our community'. At the same time HIV/AIDS service organizations, whether statutory or voluntary, have too often found themselves trapped within ideologies of integration and homogeneity, a 'colour/cultural-blind' policy, of ignorance of the psycho-social dynamics of different communities, of racism and cultural denial, of an unwillingness to challenge themselves.

Defining Needs

In the current climate of funding restrictions for work in the arena of HIV/ AIDS, many decisions are being made on the basis of epidemiological data. Several questions, though, arise concerning the value of such data in determining need and thus of funding decisions. If one looks at the statistics of AIDS cases in the United Kingdom, those defined as Asian/oriental reflect a relatively small proportion: 1.7 per cent.[3] Since ethnic minorities represent some 5.5 per cent of the population in the UK, and south Asians 52 per cent of this total, it would seem at first sight that south Asians reflect the lowest risk. World AIDS patterns must be taken into account, however: it was white people and those from sub-Saharan Africa who were the first to show signs of AIDS. Those from south and west Asia are recent partners to the epidemic, and in India AIDS was first diagnosed in the late 1980s. We suspect this will also reflect the pattern in our communities in the UK, and expect growing numbers of people from our communities to be diagnosed with AIDS in the next few years. Studies conducted by the NAZ Project have determined that male members of our communities, in particular, exhibit high levels of male-to-male sex, extra and pre-marital sex, as well as significant and growing levels of drug use. In other words, our research, which includes the socio-cultural analysis that constructs such sexual and other risky behaviours, indicates that members of our communities are at risk, and highly vulnerable to HIV infection (Khan, 1991, 1994b).

As for services, host country providers *may* recognize the implications of racism in their service development and attempt to redress the balance, but this will often be done in the context of the global 'Other'. Cultural diversity is ignored, cultural specificity lost. A service provider may intend to extend services to the 'Asian community'. But which community? And which group within this 'Asian community'? In reaching out to our communities, service providers often undertake a 'needs assessment'. They speak to the more visible, the 'community leaders' and the 'religious leaders', and they depend upon these 'spokespersons' to make known the HIV/AIDS needs of their communities. However, such leaders will too often deny any such need because they must maintain the fiction of a very moral community, free of pre-marital, extra-marital, drug using, homosexual behaviours. So who represents the HIV/AIDS needs of our communities? It is important to explore these issues of public statements and private practice.

There are also many who do not identify with their community of origin, but this does not mean that they therefore have good access to the services of the host community. As with any other community, some members of our communities exhibit traits of sexism, sexophobia and homophobia. How have these agencies and individuals been challenged around these issues? What training support has been offered, and who does the training? Some agencies will recognize this 'gatekeeping' and attempt to bypass it through sexual behaviour research, but how are the questions framed? Who is doing the research? What dynamics operate? Is it community-based and culturally appropriate?

Barriers to Access

Reliance upon the language, culture and religious framework of the host community has often precluded the taking up of HIV/AIDS education, prevention and support of services offered by many statutory and voluntary agencies. The information that *has* been presented to our communities has often been inappropriate in context and language, and lacking in understanding. Assumptions have been made about the dynamics of our behaviour, and myths have been developed and accepted (often including by members of our own communities) around arranged marriages, homophobia, religious fundamentalism, sexual behaviours and identities, extended family support systems, oppression of women, and so on. Thus it is often assumed that our communities in general, and specific groups and individuals within them, are 'hard to reach' or 'don't need HIV/AIDS services', and even that 'they cannot be educated around these issues'. This forms one aspect of racism.

Far too seldom do funding strategies, policy development and service delivery engage seriously with issues of racism and cultural diversity: services are planned and developed with the host community in mind. A gay men's sexual health promotion campaign assumes that 'gay'-identified men from ethnic minority communities have the same social and behavioural dynamics as those of 'white' gay men. A women's only service assumes that women from other communities will also use the service, but what if the woman comes from a Muslim community? Or is of a Hindu faith? Or does not speak English? Or is an Irish woman? The pre-test/post-test counselling provided by HIV testing centres and clinics is assumed to be appropriate to all those being tested, but what if the person comes from a different culture where such counselling dynamics are not only inappropriate, but unknown? What terms exist in different languages for sexuality, gender, sexual behaviours, identities? What about medical care and treatment? What about nutritional needs? What about grieving, death and dying, burial customs, last rites? What about adoption and respite care?

Because of inappropriate socio-cultural frameworks and availability of services, many people from our communities who may be at risk of HIV/STD infections do not go for testing. Too often they may learn of their HIV/AIDS status only after they have become ill. Using such services renders people visible, even if only in a restricted sense, and such visibility is felt to be dangerous by members of ethnic minority communities, risking shame and dishonour to their families.

Culturally Appropriate Services

Goodwill is in many instances nowhere near enough to ensure that service delivery is culturally appropriate. Constructions of community identities are also configured by *religious beliefs* and public practice. HIV/AIDS education, prevention and support are closely related to socially sensitive and taboo issues around sexual behaviours and practices. Such public discussions can be perceived as a threat to communities that are religiously and culturally defined. Religiosity, of any religion, especially in its orthodox forms, acts to deny behaviours perceived as being against the religious codes. Such denials are a public event, where community honour and sanctity must be seen to be maintained, and such processes need to be understood and recognized when developing appropriate services and programmes.

In developing support services for people living with HIV/AIDS, what measure of understanding exists of the *differing frameworks of identities* within our communities? Terms like 'heterosexual', 'homosexual', 'bisexual', and the identities and lifestyles that are presumed to go with them are often of very little relevance. How is this dealt with in forming support groups, be-friending services, home visits, and so on? Have differing family structures, networks, and interfamily relationships been taken on board by service providers? Have differing dietary needs, different personal and family customs been integrated into these forms of service delivery?

Issues of *language* configure the process. For many of our communities appropriate terminology in which to talk about AIDS, sex, and drug use, for example, do not exist. Where they do, they are often problematic. The same words may have different meanings for different communities. Sometimes terms may be abusive and negative, so translations may actually increase stigmatization for certain individuals and groups. Who does the translation is an issue that must be addressed with sensitivity.

The *location* of services can also have a major impact on service utilization. Honour, shame, visibility, identity, how the place is perceived, the attitudes and language of front-line staff, the posters displayed, the colour of facilities, all create an environment which may be inappropriate to people from differing communities. Who designs, decides and implements such things, and how are these decisions taken?

Finally, *access to funding* is also bound within prescriptive frameworks.

The way in which funding of resources and services are often structured means that our communities are further disempowered. Applications for funding are to be written only in the accepted form of the host language, and structured in specific ways. Monitoring data is to be collected in specific ways. Analysis is culturally defined by the host culture. Equity is thus limited to those who have access to specific value systems that are defined by the host culture.

Responses

The fact that community-based AIDS service organizations have emerged from within the minority ethnic groups themselves is testimony to the double-edged fight the early pioneers have had to conduct in order to establish support for people living with AIDS, both within British society and within the minority ethnic community itself. In the case of both the south Asian and Irish communities, community-based organizations have developed in response to their special needs in respect to HIV and AIDS.

Positively Irish Action on AIDS (PIAA): Oonagh O'Brien

Positively Irish Action on AIDS, a community-based initiative based in London, was established in 1989 to offer support and advice to Irish people affected by HIV. From the early days of the project, the sheer numbers of Irish people living with HIV who approached the project ensured that the bulk of work carried out has been around support and care, and secondary prevention. PIAA works with a mixed group of service users, including men, women and children. The population using PIAA's services have a wide range of identities and experiences, including men who have sex with men, men who identify as gay, heterosexual men and women, women with a history of injecting drug use, or who are partners of injecting drug users, and women with no contact with injecting drug use. Additionally PIAA sees a small but consistent number of black Irish people as well as women who identify as lesbians. At any one time about half of PIAA's service users have children. A number of those with children are men who identify as gay, who were in heterosexual relationships prior to, or simultaneous to, having sex with men. Additionally, a proportion of men who identify as gay have a history of injecting drug use, in some cases directly related to the problems of being gay in a Catholic and conservative culture.

An initial assessment of needs is conducted with a client worker, after which clients are referred on to appropriate mainstream services, with the support and advocacy of the client workers at PIAA. This has proved a successful method of working with limited funds, and has ensured that workers in British HIV services are supported in their work with Irish clients.

Secondary prevention has been a major focus of PIAA's work. For some injecting drug users diagnosed HIV positive for many years, there have been few opportunities to discuss safer sex. Continuity of contact with services is a problem because of the high mobility of many Irish drug users between Ireland and England. Drug users out of contact with services are vulnerable to returning to street use, and putting themselves in danger of ill health and others in danger of HIV infection.

The strongly Catholic education experienced by most Irish people has left behind a legacy of guilt and for many an inability to deal with issues of sex and sexuality. Until recently, sex has not been openly discussed in Ireland, and access to contraception has been, and still is in some areas, highly problematic. Ireland was the last country in the EU to legalize consensual sex between adult men in June 1993. It is essential for gay men who have taken many years to come to terms with their sexuality — or who may never have come to terms with it, but who have simply left Ireland as a way of dealing with the issue — to have the option of approaching services where this is understood. PIAA sees a number of older, extremely isolated gay men, who would never approach gay services, or mainstream HIV services in London, perceiving them to be for a different type of person than themselves.

Response from The Naz Project: Shivananda Khan

The Naz Project, an HIV/AIDS and Sexual Health agency working with the south Asian,[4] Turkish, Arab and Irani communities, was established in 1991 in response to the expressed need of a number of people from our communities unable to gain access to a range of services provided at the time. These included language, religion, appropriate care and befriending. For example, a 'client' who was Muslim and living with AIDS was consistently being sent pork as part of a 'meals on wheels service' provided by the local government. His first language was Urdu, and the service could not provide trained interpreters, or suitable help for a man who, while being a man who had sex with men, was also married and had children. A voluntary agency could provide an appropriate befriender and counsellor.

Recognizing the various psycho-social dynamics, Naz has developed a range of culturally appropriate programmes. These include:

- community education: to highlight awareness of HIV/AIDS, STDs and sexual health within our communities;

- male sexual health: working amongst sexually active men to promote safer sex behaviour, and to look at gender roles;
- women's sexual health: working with women in terms of gender roles, sexual behaviours and safer sex; and
- client support services: enabling access to translators, interpreters and community-based counsellors and providing a range of support groups and befriending services that are culturally and linguistically appropriate.

The specific shape and model of programmes arose from an extensive analysis of behaviours and the psycho-social dynamics within our communities, including sexual behaviour research. From these assessments we have been able to develop more appropriate health-promotion frameworks. We work in a range of community languages, and we develop a range of culturally and linguistically appropriate education and prevention resources. We also provide training and consultancy, both for our own communities and for statutory and voluntary agencies.

The Way Forward

Taking into account the issues raised in this chapter, concerning the risks of assuming a community is homogenous, and the importance of approaching the relevant personnel in communities to take on HIV/AIDS work, the following is a summary of recommendations for the development of culturally appropriate HIV/AIDS service development for migrants and ethnic minorities.

Discrimination should be challenged at all levels, both within and outside our own communities. Further, all agencies, including voluntary organizations working in the field of HIV/AIDS, sexuality and drug use should integrate discussions of racism, culture and religion into training for their staff and volunteers. Funding agreements for all such agencies should include statements and policies against homophobia, sexism, classism and discrimination, with ways of implementing and monitoring these policies specified.

A *long-term commitment* must be made to providing culturally specific services appropriate to minority ethnic communities. This requires a two-pronged approach:

1 ensuring that mainstream HIV services and all relevant statutory and voluntary agencies are sensitive to the needs of the particular minority ethnic groups using their services; and
2 supporting initiatives which develop from within the community (with safeguards concerning the issues raised in this chapter).

The latter have an important function in assuring that minority ethnic people have access to services, in developing appropriate services, and in raising awareness through training and sharing of grass-roots expertise. The major responsibility, however, must come from mainstream host-country statutory and voluntary agencies working in the field. A long-term commitment to this combined approach will help ensure that appropriate services are available and accessible for members of minority ethnic groups who are HIV positive, and greatly increase the likelihood that they are reached by prevention messages. This requires a commitment from funding bodies so that advance planning can be done, and initiatives sustained.

Educational and *preventive campaigns* on HIV/AIDS and 'safer-sex', drug use and safer needle use, with appropriate images and text, should be developed. Such resources should be targeted to specific subgroups within our communities as identified by grass-roots expertise, addressing, for example, minority ethnic people of different ages and both sexes, as well as those who have different sexual behaviours, and include men who have sex with men. They should also address varying levels of literacy in specific languages as well as in English. General campaigns often have low (if not negative) results. Specific and targeted strategies have a higher degree of encouraging awareness and behaviour change.

It is urgent that a whole range of *resources and services* be developed for people from our communities living with HIV/AIDS, and their families and partners. Such services include support groups, specialized and culture-appropriate counselling, advice, information, referral systems, and community-based befrienders, who have in-depth knowledge of the language, culture and religion of their particular 'friend'. Whilst some community-specific organizations are addressing this issue, it should also be part of the service provision of generic agencies. Programmes should include religious-specific pastoral care, culturally appropriate diets, linguistic and culture-specific counselling and support, access to linguistically appropriate literature, and access to interpreters and translators. All agencies providing HIV/AIDS education, prevention and support, whether community-based, culture specific, generic, voluntary or statutory should be effectively monitored for their development and provision of services to ethnic minority communities.

Effective models of *peer evaluation* of local community-based HIV/AIDS services should be developed in order to effectively respond to the concerns sometimes expressed that such organizations do not have the skills, knowledge and expertise to provide services dealing with such sensitive issues as sexual behaviours and injecting drug use. This could be achieved through participation in the monitoring process of those culture-specific HIV/AIDS agencies recognized for the quality of their work.

Staff of local, regional and national authorities, such as social workers, housing officers, health visitors, hospital staff and prison workers, must be *trained* in drug use, sexuality issues and HIV/AIDS within minority ethnic communities. Training in HIV/AIDS awareness for professionals from our own communities in the fields of health and social services should also be increased. In addition, there must be effective and appropriate education for our community and religious leaders, as for community-based organizations working within our communities. More people from our communities should be employed in mainstream agencies rather than being placed in marginalized 'specialist' posts. This does not invalidate the need for specialist posts, but the issues that cause this need to arise should be made part of the agendas of posts within any specific agency.

The issues of developing appropriate and accessible services around HIV and AIDS for minority ethnic communities clearly need to be urgently addressed. Approaching community 'leaders' is not enough. Too often they act as 'gatekeepers' and block the transmission of information. In developing appropriate prevention strategies that are culturally specific it must be recognized that a concern with cultural 'sensitivity' is often used as an excuse for doing nothing, for *not* addressing issues. Appropriate individuals and organizations must be encouraged, facilitated and provided adequate resources within our communities for developing their own AIDS service organizations.

Europe is culturally diverse. As citizens and residents we have the right to appropriate services. A right to challenge all forms of racism at whatever level. We are asking our basic human rights. No more and no less.

Notes

1 As recent Irish migrants migrate predominantly to England, the figures used here are not for the whole of the UK, but England only.
2 PHLS AIDS Centre-1995; Ireland, Department of Health.
3 PHLS AIDS Centre, 1995.
4 The term 'south Asian' reflects the geo-political region of the Indian subcontinent: that is, the countries of India, Pakistan, Bangladesh, Sri Lanka and Nepal.

References

AL-KHAYYAT, S. (1990) *Honour and Shame: Women in Modern Iraq*, London: Saqi Books.
ALLEN, T.W. (1994) *The Invention of the White Race. Vol. One: Racial Oppression and Social Control*, London: Verso.
BOUHDIBA, A. (1985) *Sexuality in Islam*, translated by Sheridan, A., London: Routledge & Kegan Paul.
DEPARTMENT OF HEALTH, IRELAND (1995) AIDS Statistics, March 1995.
FANON, F. (1970) *Black Skin, White Masks*, London: Paladin Books.

GREENSLADE, L. (1991) 'White skins white masks: Mental illness and the Irish in Britain', conference paper, available from Institute of Irish Studies, University of Liverpool, UK.

HARINGEY PUBLICATIONS (1991) *An Agenda for Change: Equal Opportunities, The Irish Dimension*, London: London Borough of Haringey.

HELMAN, C. (1990) *Culture, Health and Illness*, London: Wright Press.

HICKMAN, M. (1995) 'The Irish in Britain: Racism, incorporation and identity', *Irish Studies Review*, **10**, pp. 16–19.

HICKMAN, M. and WALTER, B. (1995) 'Deconstructing whiteness: Irish women in Britain', *Feminist Review*, **50**, pp. 5–19.

IRISH FEMINIST REVIEW (1984) Dublin, Ireland: Woman's Community Press.

KHAN, S. (1991) 'KHUSH: A report on the needs of south Asian lesbians and gay men in the UK', London: Naz Publications.

KHAN, S. (Ed.) (1994a) *History of Alternate Sexualities in South Asia*, a report on a three day seminar, New Delhi, India: Naz Publications.

KHAN, S. (1994b) *Contexts, Race, Culture and Sexuality: A Report and Needs Assessment on South Asian Communities*, London: Naz Publications.

KHAN, S. (1995) *Conference Report: Emerging Gay Identities in India: Implications for Sexual Health*, New Delhi, India: Naz Publications.

MANE, M. and SHUBHADA, A. (1992) *AIDS Prevention: The Socio-cultural Context in India*, Bombay: Tata Institute of Social Sciences.

O'BRIEN, O. (1993) *Assessing the Impact of HIV on the Irish Community in Britain*, London: Positively Irish Action on AIDS.

O'FLYNN, E. (1991) 'Under Piccadilly's neon: Irish and homelessness in London', London Piccadilly Advice Centre.

O'MEACHAIR, G., BURNS, A. and CLARKE, N. (1988) *Irish Homelessness: The Hidden Dimension*, London: CARA.

PARKER, A. (1992) *Nationalisms and Sexualities*, London: Routledge.

PHLS AIDS (1995) Centre-Communicable Disease Surveillance Centre and Scottish Centre for Infection and Environmental Health, unpublished Quarterly Surveillance Tables, March 1995.

PREVENTION OF TERRORISM ACT RESEARCH AND WELFARE ASSOCIATION (1995) *Statistical Update*, 17 August, Birmingham, UK.

RAFTERY, J., JONES, D. and ROSATO, M. (1990) 'The mortality of first and second generation Irish immigrants in the UK', *Social Science and Medicine*, **31**, pp. 577–84.

RACE RELATIONS ACT 1976 (1976) London: HMSO.

RATTI, R. (Ed.) (1993) *A Lotus of Another Colour*: Boston: Alyson Publications.

RIORDAN, S. (1994) *Evaluating a Community-Based Initiative: The Drugs and Irish Mobility Project*, London: Positively Irish Action on AIDS.

SABATIER, R. (1988) *Blaming Others: Prejudice, Race and Worldwide AIDS*, London: Panos.

SHARMA, S.K. (1989) *Hijras: The Labelled Deviants*, New Delhi: Gian Publishing House.

TAYLOR, S. (1990) 'Specialist services for the Irish in Britain', in *The Irish and HIV Conference Report*, London: Positively Irish Action on AIDS.

Chapter 8

HIV/AIDS Prevention Programmes for Migrants and Ethnic Minorities in Europe:
A Challenge for Policy Makers, NGOs and Health Educators

Rinske van Duifhuizen

HIV prevention programmes cannot be effective if they stigmatize a population or parts of a population. Stigmatization may be prevented if minority ethnic communities are closely involved in the development of AIDS programmes, and involving the communities also increases chances that acceptable and appropriate strategies will be developed. This starting point will serve as a recurrent theme throughout this chapter on HIV/AIDS prevention programmes for migrants and ethnic minorities in Europe.

Increasing mobility has consequences for the transmission of HIV. People from regions with low HIV-prevalence are moving to countries with high HIV-prevalence, and vice versa. People with different social and cultural backgrounds, as well as different levels of education, come into contact with each other. This mobility may have a negative impact on HIV-prevalence rates, and consequently gives rise to the necessity to increase HIV/AIDS prevention activities involving both host and mobile populations. One measure that is not considered justifiable in order to prevent the transmission of HIV is the imposition of travel and immigration restrictions. Mandatory testing for arriving migrants is impractical, ineffective, wasteful, discriminating, costly and harmful (Curtis, 1991). No screening programme for migrants can prevent the introduction and further spread of HIV infection (WHO, 1994).

Worldwide, it is becoming more and more clear that HIV is affecting those segments of the population whose human rights and dignity are least respected, people who are already living in the margins of society (Mann, 1995). In the United States as well as in Europe, the epidemic has shifted more and more towards ethnic minorities, drug users and women. Migrants and ethnic minorities should be considered as groups with specific needs for

HIV/AIDS prevention and care. Those who are most at risk for acquiring HIV in migrant communities are often also marginalized within their own communities. Those living with HIV/AIDS often experience double or even triple stigma, marginalized both within the host country and within their own community. As AIDS may increasingly be used as an argument in the discrimination against migrants and ethnic minorities, discussing the subject of HIV/AIDS and migrants requires a tactful, serious and responsible approach.

Specific HIV/AIDS Programmes for Migrants and Ethnic Minorities in Europe

In most European countries, national HIV/AIDS prevention programmes aimed at the so-called 'general public' began in 1985. Specific prevention programmes addressing migrants and ethnic minorities, however, started three or four years later, if at all. Government-sponsored general AIDS prevention activities for migrants tended to take a top–down approach. Migrants as such were not considered a risk group, however, but rather a part of the population that needed specific attention in order to be reached with relevant information. Like all inhabitants of a country, migrants have the right to be informed about HIV/AIDS, but in order to be able to reach them appropriately, approaches need to be culture-, as well as language-specific (Haour-Knipe, 1992, 1994).

The Importance of NGOs and CBOs

Fortunately, in many European countries, community-based organizations (CBOs) have taken the responsibility for and have initiated HIV/AIDS prevention activities at an early stage, sometimes under very difficult circumstances, both in their relations with the general health services, and within the communities themselves. A large variety of organizations and individuals have implemented interesting and valuable initiatives. As CBOs are the ones with grass-roots knowledge, and who have respect of the various communities, without their input no effective programme can be implemented.

The Role of Migrants Living with HIV/AIDS

In community involvement, it is extremely important to include those who are most affected: migrants and ethnic minorities living with HIV/AIDS, as well as their families, partners and friends. The beginning of the AIDS pandemic was marked by a great deal of denial within minority ethnic communities: HIV-prevalence was low, they were unable to identify with existing campaigns and programmes, and AIDS was often associated with certain forms of 'immoral behaviour' not formally tolerated in their cultures. The first cases of HIV/AIDS with ethnic communities were often kept a secret or, when it became apparent that a person was infected, they were isolated and faced severe discrimination both within and outside their own communities. Only recently have members of minority ethnic communities living with HIV/ AIDS openly addressed their fellow community members. This often has an enormous impact on the people concerned, bringing the realities of the pandemic very close (Deutsch AIDS-Hilfe, 1993).

So far, only a few prevention programmes aimed at migrants and ethnic minorities have focused on the aspects of solidarity and support for people living with HIV/AIDS. Most of the activities have been focused on the primary prevention of HIV-infection. Just as in general population campaigns, however, aspects of prevention and solidarity need to be included in HIV/ AIDS programmes for migrants and ethnic minorities.

The Necessity of a Two-sided Approach

Both 'top–down' and 'bottom–up' approaches should be implemented so that they can reinforce and complement each other. Attention given to ethnic minorities and HIV/AIDS at the decision-making and policy levels should be interlinked with that within community-based structures of the migrants themselves. National AIDS Programmes should involve and consult migrant communities and, at the same time, they should stimulate and support initiatives within these communities. This can be done by providing technical assistance (in writing proposals, budgeting, etc.), by encouraging networking, and by sharing relevant information. Regular consultation involving community-based organizations of migrants and ethnic minorities will greatly improve the effectiveness of the programmes developed. A useful tool for CBOs is the acknowledgment by national AIDS programmes that 'migrants and ethnic minorities' have been identified as a priority group. This is particularly useful in lobbying at the local level.

Existing Programmes Today

Within the European region there are numerous differences, in migrant populations, immigration policies, HIV/AIDS epidemiology, health policies, economic situations, HIV/AIDS networks and so on. There is also a multitude of cultural, language and religious differences. Only a few national governments have taken on the responsibility of developing and supporting interventions, focusing on these specific groups on national and local levels.

Western/Northern Europe

The countries of western and northern Europe have relatively high HIV-prevalence rates, comprehensive national AIDS programmes, and quite sophisticated health-care systems. This part of Europe has been active in the fight against AIDS from the beginning of the pandemic. Both governmental and non-governmental structures are closely involved in HIV/AIDS policies, and programmes for the general population and specific target groups.

The Netherlands, Norway, Switzerland and the United Kingdom were among the first to identify 'migrants and ethnic minorities' as a priority group. Specific activities have been undertaken in these countries since 1989, all of them stressing the right to information for the entire population of a country. The implementation of programmes in these countries, however, varies greatly. In the United Kingdom for example, numerous AIDS-service organizations (ASOs) for minority ethnic communities arose. Some work at a national level, others at a local level. Examples are Blackliners, Black HIV/ AIDS Network, the Naz-Project, and Positively Irish Action on AIDS. In Norway, The Netherlands and Switzerland, on the other hand, migrant-specific AIDS service organizations have either been absent in the fight against AIDS or created only recently, and are closely linked with health authorities and governmental structures.

In many western European countries, however, there is no national coordinating body for HIV/AIDS programmes for migrants and ethnic minorities. In Germany, it was not until 1995 that a national coordination project was started. This certainly does not imply that there is nothing happening in these countries, but the activities are *ad hoc*, poorly funded, and the organizations are working in relative isolation.

Southern Europe

The countries of southern Europe tend to have high HIV-prevalence rates, they have reasonably good health services and national AIDS programmes. However, there are only a few experiences in non-governmental responses to HIV/AIDS. Countries such as Greece, Italy, Spain and Portugal have attracted immigration only recently, as a result of economic and political developments. Only a few years ago, these countries were still considered as 'sending countries'. Issues around migrants, ethnic minorities and refugees are relatively new in this region, and HIV/AIDS is certainly not a priority on their agendas. Although more NGOs are becoming involved in HIV/AIDS, only a few of them take into account the needs of migrants and ethnic minorities.

In some southern European countries, epidemiological data is now beginning to alert policy makers, providing them with arguments to include migrants and ethnic minorities in their work in order to protect their own native population. Although ASOs and migrants' organizations may certainly benefit from this development, it is a dangerous starting point when talking about health promotion in general, and HIV/AIDS prevention in particular. There is a risk that the approach will be stigmatizing, and it does not allow migrant organizations to become appropriately involved.

Central and Eastern Europe

The countries of central and eastern Europe are characterized by low HIV-prevalence rates, relatively poor medical services, AIDS programmes that hardly reach the general public, and a lack of non-governmental organizations involved in HIV/AIDS. Since the liberalization of travel restrictions between eastern and western Europe in 1990, mobility and migration in this region has drastically increased. Although the HIV-prevalence in this region is still very low compared with the rest of Europe, the increased mobility to and from this region holds serious potential for the increase of infectious diseases, including HIV. It is only recently that NGOs, including some AIDS service organizations, have been created in this region.

In this region there are several specific mobile populations (e.g. Roma and Sinti), and several serious ethnic conflicts. So far, HIV/AIDS is low on the agenda of policy makers in general. And migrants and refugees do not figure at all on the agendas of the small number of ASOs in this region. However, other NGOs (e.g. the Red Cross) are now slowly beginning to take into account the sexual health issues of migrants and ethnic minorities.

Why Did or Do Countries (Still) not Deal with the Issue?

The main reasons for *not* starting to develop specific programmes from the beginning of the epidemic include fear of stigmatization, the existence of so-called integration policies, and the size of migrant groups. The 'excuse' most often given for not doing anything in the field of HIV/AIDS prevention for migrants and ethnic minorities is the fear of stigmatization and discrimination. This fear is often intensified by a lack of skills and experience in working with and for migrants, or ethnic communities in general. If migrants and ethnic minorities themselves are closely involved in the development and implementation of prevention programmes, however, stigmatization can be prevented.

At the same time, the so-called 'integration policies' in many European countries result in less, or even no support for community-based migrant organizations, minority ethnic media, and social services. Structures and networks are further limited as a result of recent budget cuts: support for these organizations no longer seems to fit into local and national policies. While in most European countries, the number of 'immigrants' does not exceed 6 per cent overall, there may be substantial concentrations (20 per cent or more) in large cities, and in certain areas within these cities (Muus, 1993). An enormous variety of minority ethnic communities may be present. This makes it more difficult to implement HIV prevention activities, both from a logistical and a financial perspective. Nonetheless, such groups have the right to be informed about HIV/AIDS. However, ethnic minorities often disappear into the gaps between prevention and intervention programmes, which may lead to potential exposure to risk, due to lack of information and health care.

Approaches

Although the circumstances certainly are not ideal, and the possibilities of establishing AIDS prevention programmes for migrants and ethnic minorities vary greatly from country to country, much useful experience has been gained. We can distinguish programmes oriented toward individuals (e.g. minority ethnic hotlines), groups (e.g. training minority ethnic people as educators to organize group sessions), and the mass media (minority ethnic radio, television and newspapers). Furthermore, educational materials play an important supporting role in AIDS prevention programmes, and involvement of the target group in all phases of the prevention strategy is crucial.

An Individual Approach: Ethnic Minority AIDS Hotlines

Various countries have initiated hotlines in different languages. These vary, from oral messages (audio-cassettes) to a regular personal service, and may include hotline campaigns over a limited period of time (e.g. on World AIDS

Day). A hotline is one of the most appropriate channels by which to offer anonymous and individual counselling, but manpower and finance is not always available.

Hotlines for Turks and Moroccans were launched as an experiment in The Netherlands in 1991 as part of the National AIDS Helpline. Twice a week (one evening and one afternoon) people could call these hotlines with personal questions about HIV/AIDS. Turkish and Moroccan men and women were trained as counsellors, and became part-time paid employees. There was an extensive publicity campaign, including the ethnic media available for Turks and Moroccans living in The Netherlands. After two years, the service was evaluated. There were several differences in comparison with Dutch callers to the national AIDS helpline: only 20 per cent of the callers were female, the average duration of the calls was longer (±10 minutes), there were more so-called 'basic questions' (about transmission, symptoms, etc.) and there were more questions about other health issues and problems. Although the average number of calls was only one per hour, this is a relatively high number, considering the limited hours of service and the small size of the target populations. Although the hotlines for Turks and Moroccans certainly fulfilled the need for information, the evaluation concluded that the experiment was too expensive: the cost per call exceeded Dfl. 150 (US$ 90). The Turkish and Arabic hotlines now only operate live during short-term campaigns, e.g. around World AIDS Day and linked to some television programmes. During the rest of the year, callers can listen to a taped message.

Before planning a hotline service, one should clearly consider the logistics and costs likely to be involved. In order to have a successful hotline service, there should be appropriate publicity on a regular basis, e.g. by using posters and leaflets, and by placing advertisements in specific ethnic media (written press, radio and television). In evaluation, the results and costs of a specialist hotline are often compared with similar initiatives for the population as a whole. However, when a specific target group is considered a priority, for example because they are especially vulnerable, or because they are living in a disadvantaged position, extra costs should be allowed in order to reach the group, to overcome lack of knowledge and so on.

Group Education Approaches

Group education is especially relevant when working with minority ethnic communities, preferably when it takes place in their own language and is arranged by their own people as counsellors. This way, people appear to find it easier to express themselves about especially sensitive issues, they have the possibility of exchanging ideas and experiences, and of supporting one another within the group. Moreover, many non-western cultures have a less individualistic tradition of dealing with problems and delicate issues. A group approach may therefore fit better into the culture. Often, it may be useful to conduct such education in single sex groups.

In several European countries, members of migrant communities have been trained as peer educators, outreach workers and counsellors. For example a Moroccan woman gives information to other Moroccan women visiting a health clinic in Brussels. Turkish men are visiting organizations, mosques and coffee shops in Amsterdam, in order to talk about sexual health with groups of other Turkish men. A Colombian man is organizing a self-help group for Spanish-speaking migrants living with HIV/AIDS in Berlin. Examples of some group education strategies implemented in Switzerland are discussed in Chapter 9 of this volume.

Group education can be organized by paid workers or by volunteers. For the intervention to be effective, it is essential that a peer educator be reliable and professional. Regular training therefore needs to be provided, and educators should be kept informed about any relevant developments or new materials. Evaluation of the group meetings may provide information to facilitate further develop of the programme. It not only provides information about the number of people that were reached, but also about the needs of a community (both AIDS-specific needs and needs relating to broader health and social issues). It provides more insight into specific cultural and religious aspects (e.g. traditional healing, condom use) and into the extent to which the materials used were appreciated, as well as, for example, the response of the minority ethnic press.

Use of Ethnic Mass Media

The ethnic media play an essential role in providing information to migrant communities. Migrants and ethnic minorities often use different media than that of the host population. In many European countries, there are radio stations in the languages of the main ethnic minorities. These media may originate in the country of origin, or may have been established by migrant communities in the host country. They include journals and magazines, but also radio and television programmes. There are, for example, a large number of Turkish and Arabic television programmes available in Europe through satellite television. An enormous number of people can be reached by making use of the ethnic mass media for information about HIV/AIDS. Such media are especially suitable for reaching the people who do not participate in group meetings or other such activities. They provide on excellent opportunity for setting the agenda, and creating a climate within communities that will later facilitate communication about a taboo issue.

The diversity of the available media may create some confusion, however. Information diffused in the countries of origin does not always contain the same messages as that in the host countries. Articles containing incorrect information in Turkish newspapers, for example, once caused a deluge of worried callers to the AIDS hotline for Turks in The Netherlands. It is important to collaborate with the media in countries of origin, and work where possible with the same messages, for example, to strengthen and to support each other's initiatives.

In 1995, a European initiative was funded by the European Commission called 'Translating the AIDS message across Europe'. It was initiated by Social Action Radio and BBC World Services. In close collaboration with the national AIDS helplines in France, Italy and The Netherlands, radio programmes were developed in the languages of several minority ethnic communities, such as in Arabic and Turkish. The programmes referred to AIDS helplines. Local minority ethnic radio stations in the different countries were contacted so that the programmes could be broadcast before and during World AIDS Day. Unfortunately, migrant organizations were insufficiently involved in the project to bring broader integration of the campaign with other prevention activities.

In 1992, the Health Education Authority in England designed a mass media campaign aimed at the four largest ethnic minority communities in the country: Asians, south east Asians, Afro-Caribbeans and people from Middle Eastern countries. The campaign included posters and leaflets (in eight different languages), and it involved the black and minority ethnic press and community radio. Various organizations were informed in advance about the campaign so that they were able to organize complementary activities. The campaign was evaluated and received many positive reactions. The general impression was that the media that were used had been appropriate.

Ethnic minority media need to be included whenever an HIV or AIDS campaign is started. They should be put on mailing lists for press releases and kept informed about relevant developments. If necessary, a training package should be developed, in order to enable the media to produce their own programmes and articles about HIV and AIDS.

Other Innovative Approaches

Many different methods of implementing AIDS prevention strategies for migrants and ethnic minorities have proved useful, including music and theatre.

A group of Cape-Verdian musicians and performers from Portugal and The Netherlands have developed a performance about HIV/AIDS in the Cape-Verdian community. All of them received training about HIV/AIDS. After a pilot phase, the project was implemented in other European countries. The group visited several Cape-Verdian community centres in Lisbon, Luxembourg, Brussels and Paris to perform the theatre play and the songs about HIV/AIDS. The play was adapted to the audience present each time it was performed. After the play, the musicians and players stayed on in order to answer questions and provide more information. Furthermore, leaflets and an audio-cassette with some songs were distributed. In Switzerland, a group of Latin-American performers implemented a similar initiative (see Chapter 9).

The London-based NAZ Project is offering HIV prevention workshops that make use of traditional Indian dances and music. 'Insight into life' is a one-day practical workshop meant for exploring the impact of HIV/AIDS upon diverse communities. By using dance and theatre, and by means of participative learning, the workshop aims at developing a greater awareness of these issues. As a supplement to the workshop, a performance has been developed, enabling participants to use the knowledge gained in the workshop to further explore the issues.

Development of Appropriate Educational Materials

It is essential to develop materials for further information to support education and prevention activities and programmes. Various materials can be distinguished: written/printed materials (leaflets, posters, etc.), audio materials (radio commercials, audio-cassettes), and audio-visual materials such as series of slides and video programmes. For the development of appropriate materials, it is important that the intended audience be involved. They are the ones who should define the needs to be taken into account.

Many people find it easier to understand the spoken word than written material. In different societies, the arts have been used to educate people or to introduce new ideas. By means of story-telling, people can understand problems more clearly, and identify their options for behaviour change. In general, audio-visual support will be much more effective than written materials for programmes for migrants. This has to do with cultural background, socio-economic position, and the available minority ethnic media in the different countries. In many migrant communities, there are problems of literacy, particularly among women. In countries of origin, it may have been common for people to receive information about various subjects by way of oral communication, mainly through family members, neighbours and, quite often, the radio.

Materials developed within the national AIDS programmes should be non-stigmatizing, and they should also offer the possibility for different communities to identify with them. Campaigns and materials for the general public should also aim to be multicultural, so that different members and communities can visually identify with the campaign. This is especially relevant for second and third generation migrants, who are usually more integrated into the host society.

At the same time, migrant community-based organizations should be given the opportunity to develop their own materials in accordance with their own culture and language. These opportunities should be supported by governmental structures, as well as by AIDS service organizations. If necessary, training in this area should be provided in order to enable migrant organizations to develop their own materials and initiate campaigns.

Members of the minority ethnic community should be involved from the start in order to be able to identify needs correctly. Members of migrant communities are very often only involved once the draft material has already been prepared, a point by which important choices have already been made. What is the use of pre-testing a leaflet if people do not want to read about AIDS, but would have preferred receiving the information on an audiocassette? Artists from migrant communities themselves should where possible be involved. Literal translations of already existing brochures should not be used, as this does not leave any space for culturally specific expressions, language and words. There are many opportunities to collaborate between countries in material development. Efforts can be pooled so as to develop common materials when a given minority ethnic community is relatively small in one country but larger in another. Materials developed in the country of origin may be useful in the host countries, as well as the other way around.

> During a European meeting, a working group of Turkish AIDS prevention workers from seven countries proposed the development of a brochure and poster to be used both for the Turkish population in Europe and in Turkey itself. It was decided that it should become an A5-sized comic book. A Turkish artist was hired to prepare the first draft, based on the story provided by the working group. The draft brochure was pre-tested in participating countries, and the working group met again to discuss the results. Although the design was very comprehensible and attractive, the story was thought to be too stereotyped and sexist, by both women and men. In order to put some humour into it, the designer had used exaggerated examples, but he changed the story and deleted several pages of the draft version. In addition to these changes, the working group also identified the

need for a more theoretical chapter, and a list of addresses for more information. Four text pages were added to the end of the brochure. Thirty-five thousand copies of the brochure have now been distributed all over Europe.

Pre-testing of educational materials is essential. It can prevent mistakes, and provides information on which materials will be appropriate, comprehensible and attractive. Pre-testing should not necessarily involve large numbers of respondents. Selecting the right people (those who properly represent the target group) is more important than the number of people. Most of the time, no additional information is gathered after ten people have been interviewed. Pre-testing can best be done in the native language of the community involved, and by a member of this community.

Common Bottlenecks in HIV/AIDS Programmes for Migrants and Ethnic Communities

Although a number of relevant programmes and experiences are already under way, there is still a long way to go and there are a number of obstacles to overcome. Not all of the problems discussed below are specific to HIV/AIDS, but all of the various issues relating to vulnerability in general are represented in this epidemic. Examples include accessibility of health care and the fact that existing networks and community-based organizations are not always made use of. Bottlenecks are frequently encountered in HIV/AIDS education programmes for migrants and ethnic minorities.

Difficulties Developing a Non-stigmatizing Approach

In order to be effective, prevention programmes must not stigmatize a population, or parts of a population. The risk of stigmatization is especially problematic in the development of national, mass media campaigns and educational materials. What can be done about it? The only way to prevent stigmatization is to involve the target group in the development of strategies from the beginning. This way, the symbols, language and images appropriate for the specific target group(s) can be used, misunderstandings can be avoided, and the messages developed will probably be acceptable and appropriate for the respective communities.

Lack of Data, Research and Evaluation

Sound policy making and planning of health promotion require better quality information, and data about the health status of minority ethnic people (Curtis, 1991). Even more information is needed to legitimize prevention and to fight common prejudices. Such data should be gathered with proper safeguards against abuse, such as measures in order to avoid discrimination of ethnic minorities and migrants. Preferably, data should be gathered by members of the communities themselves.

Lack of Mobilization in the Field and of Involvement of Community-based Organizations

HIV/AIDS should be on the agenda of migrant organizations, and migrants should be on the agenda of ASOs. Therefore, intersectoral collaboration is necessary. Initiatives should be taken at local, national and international levels in order to link these organizations and to reinforce them. Since the duplication of tasks is to be avoided, coordination is essential. Many existing channels of communication for migrant communities can be used for HIV/AIDS programmes, including those that are informal.

Lack of Support from National AIDS Programmes and Financial Resources

In many countries, ethnic minorities are not considered a specific target group, and local and national governments do not have budgets for specific HIV/AIDS programmes. Private initiatives sometimes attempt to fill this gap, but they are not always able to give sufficient help. Within national AIDS programmes a budget should be allocated for prevention and care initiatives focused on migrants and ethnic minorities. Assistance and training in project design, project management, and funding should be provided when needed.

International Networking

Since 1990, the issue of HIV/AIDS and migrants and ethnic minorities has been addressed regularly in European and international settings, and in various international meetings and publications. Some important networking has been initiated, both in the area of governmental (e.g. the annual WHO meeting of National AIDS Coordinators) and non-governmental structures (e.g. Eurocaso/Migrants Network, and within the European Project on AIDS and Mobility). Collaboration, both within Europe and with the migrants' countries of origin appeared to stimulate initiatives in different countries (see also Chapter 14, this volume).

Materials developed by a specific migrant group in one country may be adopted in another without having to repeat the whole and sometimes expensive process of development. Close collaboration with the country of origin may also strengthen the messages, and promote identification with the materials and projects. Some prevention methods and materials used in the countries of origin may also be useful when working with migrants in Europe. For example a video programme that was produced in Morocco, about a woman living with AIDS, proved to be useful in working with Moroccan immigrants in various European countries.

Efforts to stop the further spread of the AIDS epidemic should take mobility (both travel and migration) into account. Attempts to solve the HIV/AIDS problem exclusively on a national level will meet with tragically inadequate results. Increased mobility necessitates cooperation between AIDS service organizations and health authorities on a European and an international level. International networking is essential in creating awareness, promoting solidarity, exchanging models of good practice, and in strengthening local efforts in fighting AIDS.

Final Remarks and Recommendations

HID/AIDS prevention activities for migrants and ethnic minorities depend on the target group, the networks and the methods that are used. The target group 'migrants and ethnic minorities' is such a varied group of people that it is almost impossible to make general recommendations. However, both practical experiences and research findings (Haour-Knipe, 1992) demonstrate that certain factors should be taken into account when working with a migrant or a minority ethnic community.

1   It is important to respect diversity. Migrant groups differ widely, and they include top salary managers and high officials of multinational organizational as well as unskilled workers, refugees, asylum seekers and displaced persons. Within any one minority ethnic community there are many differences, e.g. of age, gender, generation and duration of stay in the host country.

2   Migrants should not be considered a risk group, but a group with specific needs regarding HIV/AIDS prevention and care programmes. In Europe, awareness about the need to provide migrants with specific HIV/AIDS projects has grown in the last few years, but it is not yet standard procedure to involve migrant communities integrally in the development of such programmes. Attempts to do so should be supported by governmental, as well as non-governmental organizations.

3   It is the responsibility of every government to inform the inhabitants of its country about significant health risks. Policies on HIV/AIDS should therefore take into account the needs of migrant populations and ethnic minority groups. In doing so issues of race and ethnicity should be discussed as well. Very often, the reason for not considering migrants as a specific target group in HIV/AIDS programmes is fear of stigmatization. However, this should not lead to failure to undertake health promotion, since it is possible to develop appropriate prevention activities without stigmatizing. Additionally, in policy development we should ensure that the needs and views of migrants and ethnic minorities are taken into account when policies are prepared; that issues of racism and discrimination are part of policy; that monitoring takes place from the migrants' and ethnic minorities' perspective; and that there is active consultation and continuing contact with representatives of different migrant groups and ethnic communities.

4   Members of ethnic communities should be represented at all levels of policy making, as well as in the implementation of HIV/AIDS programmes in order to guarantee that these programmes will really meet the needs of their communities. Involvement of the target group in all stages of the planning and implementation process will improve the quality of programmes. Indeed it is the only way to develop a successful programme.

5   Ethnic minorities themselves should not be alone in taking responsibility for the development of appropriate programmes. This responsibility should be shared by governmental authorities and the public organizations responsible for the population as a whole, including people from different ethnic backgrounds. These initiatives need to be complementary: people should be able to make their own choices for appropriate counselling, care, etc. Specific networks and/ or the minority ethnic media should be made use of in general HIV/ AIDS prevention campaigns.

6   Health promotion approaches may need to be adapted in order to reach all segments with appropriate information. Although migrants and ethnic minorities have the formal right to health care, access to these services is still problematic (Bollini, 1992). Attention to the health needs of migrants and ethnic minorities will greatly improve their access to health services.

7 As a result of the opening of the borders in central and eastern Europe and the former Soviet Union, the northern and western European countries now have to provide for new groups of migrants and ethnic minorities. So far, there is little experience in this field, rendering European cooperation essential. Priority should also be given to collaboration with countries in the former Soviet Union and central and eastern Europe, as HIV/AIDS prevalence is still low in these regions and we should make an effort to keep it as low as possible.

8 More and more initiatives for migrants and ethnic minorities are facing budget cuts as a result of so-called 'integration policies'. The growth and the increasing influence of extremist organizations all over Europe is a concern to all of us. As a result, people with HIV/AIDS as well as migrants and ethnic minorities are having to deal with a double stigma, as well as a lack of appropriate services.

Finally, it should be clear that the above eight factors are closely linked. Sound policy making is impossible without research and involvement of the community, programme developers should take political and economic factors into account, basic human rights need to be part of the policy.

The Next Step Forward: Sharing the Challenge

In order to move forward, we have to confront ourselves, our own status quo, our fears, our uncertainties . . . A new public health is dawning, devoted to dealing simultaneously with immediate needs and societal root causes . . . Connecting inner truth and global realities . . . In answering these challenges, we as policy makers, NGOs and health educators, should embed human rights issues, when fighting this epidemic and its devastating consequences. By joining expertize and knowledge to modern human rights thinking, one can learn how to simultaneously attack the root causes, and the pathological expressions of these causes, in terms of inequality in health status. AIDS is about society, more than about a virus. (Mann, 1995)

Although attention to HIV/AIDS issues related to migrants and ethnic minorities has increased in the last couple of years, there is still a long way to go, and a lot of work to be done. International mobility is now a prominent feature of virtually all societies, and HIV knows no borders. In the field of health promotion in general, and AIDS prevention in particular, there are policies and programmes to be developed in order to be able to respond appropriately to the needs of migrant communities, and of migrants living with HIV/AIDS.

Unfortunately, some governments have only recently started their activities in this field, out of fear of infection of their own native population. This is a very negative and discriminatory starting point. Every member of society has the right to be informed about HIV/AIDS, and should be enabled to protect his or her health.

Governmental organizations should acknowledge the important role ethnic minority organizations and other NGOs should play in HIV/AIDS prevention and care. Non-governmental and governmental organizations should work together to develop appropriate prevention programmes, to combat discrimination and the violation of human rights, and to develop care facilities for migrants living with HIV/AIDS. 'Shared rights: shared responsibilities', as the World Health Organization put it on World AIDS Day 1995 — a good starter for continuing our efforts to stop the further spread of HIV, and to provide support to those living with HIV/AIDS.

References

AIDS and MOBILITY (1993) *A Manual for the Implementation of Prevention Activities Aimed at Travellers and Migrants*, Amsterdam: European Project AIDS and Mobility.

AIDS and MOBILITY (1994) First European Workshop· on HIV/AIDS in Relation to Refugees and Asylum Seekers, 29 June–2 July, 1994, Noordwijkerhout, The Netherlands.

BOLLINI, P. (1992) 'Health policies for immigrant populations in the 1990s: A comparative study in seven receiving countries', *International Migration*, **30**, pp. 103–13.

BÖTTINGER, M. and ERIKSSON, G. (1993) 'Increasing impact of immigration on the HIV epidemiology in Sweden', paper given at the IXth International Conference on AIDS, Berlin.

CURTIS, H. (Ed.) (1991) *Promoting Sexual Health*, Proceeding of the Second International Workshop on Prevention of Sexual Transmission of HIV and other Sexually Transmitted Diseases, Cambridge, March 1991, London: BMA Foundation for AIDS.

DADA, M. (1992) *Multilingual AIDS, HIV Information for the Black and Minority Ethnic Communities*, London: Health Education Authority.

DEUTSCH AIDS-HILFE (Ed.) (1993) *Migrants, Ethnic Minorities and AIDS*, Documentation of the First European Meeting for the Exchange of Information, Blossin, May, 1993.

DUIFHUIZEN, R. VAN (1994) 'Migrants, ethnic minorities and HIV/AIDS: Some European experiences', paper presented in Stockholm, 11 March 1994.

HAOUR-KNIPE, M. (1992) 'Assessing AIDS prevention among migrant populations', in PACCAUD, F., VADER, J.P. and GUTZWILLER, F. (Eds) *Assessing AIDS Prevention*, pp. 171–87, Berlin: Birkhäuser.

HAOUR-KNIPE, M. (1994) 'Migrant populations; The development of something to evaluate', *Social and Preventive Medicine*, **37**, Suppl. 1, pp. S79–S94.

HAOUR-KNIPE, M. and DUBOIS-ARBER, F. (1993) 'Minorities, immigrants and HIV/AIDS epidemiology: Concerns about the use and quality of data', *European Journal of Public Health*, **3**, pp. 259–63.

MANN, J. (1995) 'The next step: AIDS, communities and human rights', presented 24 May, François-Xavier Bagnoud Center for Health and Human Rights, Boston, MA. .

MUUS, P. (1993) 'Internationale migrantie naar Europa, Een analyse van internationale migratie, migratiebeleid en mogelijkheden tot sturing van immigratie, met bijzondere aandacht voor de Europese gemeenschap en Nederland', Universiteit van Amsterdam.

PACCAUD, F., VADER, J.P. and GUTZWILLER, F. (Eds) (1990) *Assessing AIDS Prevention: Selected Papers Presented at the International Conference held in Montreux, Switzerland*, Berlin: Birkhäuser.

WORLD HEALTH ORGANIZATION (1994) Background Paper on 'Long term travel restrictions and HIV/AIDS', draft version, 22 September 1994, Geneva: WHO.

Chapter 9

A National AIDS Prevention Programme for Migrants

Didier Burgi and François Fleury

This chapter, aimed at policy-makers, describes the development and implementation of a programme grounded in a national AIDS prevention strategy, but specifically oriented towards a country's migrants and ethnic minorities. Basic principles are emphasized, as are the particular methods used to justify the programme within the national strategy and to implement it. Examples are given of the methods used to encourage communities, local authorities and relevant organizations to respond in ways adapted to the needs of the target groups.

It is assumed that, before implementation, a programme aimed at migrants and ethnic minorities must

1 be based on health principles acceptable to both local public authorities and to the targeted communities (acceptability);
2 intervene on the basis of well defined criteria, in accordance with the general objectives of the national campaign (accordance feasibility); and
3 be based on a flexible, participative method (appropriateness and involvement).

Before describing AIDS prevention activities for migrants, we will address some preliminary questions of why? and how? Our starting point will thus be with the given general framework, the Swiss AIDS Prevention Campaign and its influence on the design of work among migrants and ethnic minorities.

The Swiss National Programme for AIDS Prevention

The first national programme for AIDS prevention began in Switzerland in 1987. In harmony with the WHO 'Health 2000' programme and with recommendations by the WHO Global Programme on AIDS, it included psychological and social dimensions, and emphasized three main targets: the prevention of new cases of HIV infection; the reduction of negative effects of the epidemic; and the promotion of mutual solidarity. This is an 'integration model', based on the conviction that individuals are capable of learning, and can be motivated to adopt preventive behaviours (Dubois-Arber *et al.*, 1989). A key element is to take into account specific personal beliefs, and different ethnic and cultural backgrounds. The process underlying any change in behaviour patterns goes through the following stages:

1   During the first stage, *problem awareness* must be raised by continuous information and follow-up. Being aware of the problem and knowing the relevant risks, as well as the measures of prevention, will permit the individual to act appropriately.

2   During the next stage, *motivation* can be achieved through persuasive arguments. Social support in relevant settings can make a significant contribution here. A central point in prevention work is to make communities feel concerned about issues they might otherwise perceive as the problem of others, to cut through denial.

3   During the *skills stage*, skills should be developed to enable individuals to put their knowledge of low-risk behaviour and protective options into practice. This ability to act correctly and consistently must be encouraged through the appropriate training of health educators or mediators from minority communities.

4   During the *implementation and permanent support stage*, the process of behaviour change must be promoted consistently and repeatedly, so that behaviour patterns, once adopted, can be stabilized, and so that 'relapses' can be recognized and exploited as opportunities for further learning.

Where do migrants and ethnic minorities fit into such a strategy? Clearly, all prevention stages must be taken into account while working with migrant groups, including information for the general public, information and motivation of specific target groups, prevention and counselling for individuals. Messages at all levels must be communicated in an understandable form so as to achieve a broad effect. Certain terms used uncritically in the past cause bias and need to be redefined. Thus, in this programme, our target group of migrants is not defined by a specific pattern of behaviour, but by the need for specific modes of intervention. Finally, the need for a specific programme for non-Swiss nationals living in Switzerland is by no means to be taken as an indication that these groups are more likely to practise high risk behaviours. They may simply be more difficult to reach because of unique social, linguistic, ethnic, religious and economic characteristics. Thus promoting and implementing AIDS prevention programmes towards migrants and ethnic minorities must be part of a global programme (Fleury, 1989). It cannot be

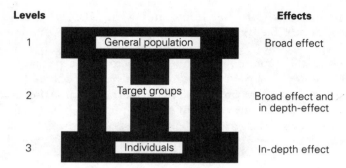

Figure 9.1 HIV/AIDS prevention activities for migrants and ethnic minorities
Source: Federal Office of Public Health, 1993

considered as 'target group work' only. HIV/AIDS prevention activities for migrants and ethnic minorities can be represented as described in Figure 9.1.

What the Policy-maker Needs to Prepare Politically Acceptable Answers

The first step, before a programme is started, is to identify the reasons for targeted intervention, to provide decision-makers with clear information and reasons for starting specific AIDS prevention measures aimed at migrants and ethnic minorities (Burgi, 1991). We attempted to respond to three basic questions.

Is the target-group well informed? The Institute of Social and Preventive Medicine of the University of Lausanne has been in charge of evaluating the Swiss national AIDS prevention strategy since 1986. As part of a large evaluation programme, among which specific target groups were examined (young people or drug users for example), a number of studies specifically assessed knowledge about routes of HIV infection, methods of protection, and attitudes towards AIDS and its prevention, among migrant groups such as seasonal workers and refugees.

These studies (Fleury, 1989, 1990, 1991; Fleury *et al.*, 1991; Haour-Knipe *et al.*, 1992; Fleury and Haour-Knipe, 1993; Haour-Knipe *et al.*, 1993) showed that, whatever the nationality of the people questioned, the main HIV transmission routes were known. Nevertheless, incorrect assumptions about AIDS transmission and protection were widespread, and considerable uncertainty was noted, for example, about such issues as the significance and purpose of the test, the existence or non-existence of a vaccine, the risk of infection when kissing or using the same cooking utensils. The data also showed that condom use during transitory sexual relations was less frequent than among

Swiss nationals of the same age. Studies showed moreover that legal status can also play a role in relationships: seasonal workers, for example, who do not have the right to family reunification during their first years in Switzerland, are more likely to have transitory relationships.

Are messages acceptable and understandable. Do they have to be adapted? Qualitative studies (Fleury, 1989) showed that even the well-known 'Stop AIDS' logo was not sufficiently clear, and was sometimes misunderstood by some ethnic minority respondents. The red coloured O, representing a condom, was misinterpreted as a red traffic light, a sign of danger or as a blood spot, for example, showing to what extent even a central message (condom use) can remain uncomprehended.

To what extent should epidemiological data play a central role in formulating specific prevention programmes aimed at migrants and ethnic minorities? Epidemiological data concerning the nationality of diagnosed AIDS cases indicates that the prevalence of AIDS among non-nationals in Switzerland is comparable to that of the general population living in the country. Nationality was known for 98 per cent of the 2228 cases of AIDS reported to the Federal Office of Public Health by the end of December 1991. Non-nationals accounted for about 21 per cent of these AIDS cases: of these 72 per cent came from other European countries, and 28 per cent from non-European countries. The number of cases of AIDS recorded in Switzerland from 1983 to 1990 per 100 000 inhabitants was twenty-two for Swiss citizens and twenty-three for persons from other European countries. No significant change has been registered since then.

Whilst important differences exist according to country of origin, AIDS case data on non-nationals by itself is not felt to be sufficient to justify targeted prevention: it is far more relevant to target behaviours which might lead to the transmission of HIV. Swiss health authorities have deliberately decided not to publish epidemiological data according to nationality in order to avoid stigmatizing specific groups, and the risk of discriminatory practices, such as mandatory HIV testing, which might be advocated by some elements of health and political systems. In specific situations, however, for instance when addressing certain community leaders, data regarding national groups may be communicated. Such information can stimulate key persons to fully grasp the scope of the problem and to become involved in preventive action. More specific information on the risk behaviour which has lead to HIV infection may be shared with the programme's collaborators.

Identifying Principles and Defining Priorities

In its conceptualization, the programme was committed to three basic principles:

1 Only the well informed can protect themselves and others against the spread of HIV and AIDS. The general population of migrants and ethnic minorities must therefore be specifically informed.

2 AIDS prevention for migrants and ethnic minorities must be based on the universal right to know rather than on any notion of specific risk. This principle derives from the first target of the WHO report 'Health for all by the year 2000' (equity in health) and the Ottawa Charter ensuring equal opportunities and resources to enable all people to achieve their fullest health potential.

3 Only a participatory, community-based, prevention programme stands a chance of being accepted and understood. The programme itself must be coordinated by people who belong to the targeted communities, and must involve as many key-persons and community peer-educators as possible.

Before the programme started, the above-mentioned reasons for implementing it were clearly explained and discussed in the communities involved. Leaders of immigrants' associations, diplomatic representatives and informal leaders were given particular attention.

Among the specific criteria determining priorities and levels of intervention were: size of national groups (numerical data); social and economic status in the host country (structural data); degree of integration in Switzerland (environmental data); degree of internal organization of the community (organizational data); and knowledge of AIDS and general evaluation of the campaign in the country of origin (problem-specific data). Other important points, particularly relevant for counselling and care, include gender, family situation, age, educational level, social status, legal status in Switzerland, religion, culture, and relation to a target group with high-risk behaviour patterns (sex workers, injecting drug users, gay men, etc.).

In addressing the needs of migrants from traditional guest-worker countries, the first concern, based on the notion of participation, was to engage AIDS coordinators to be responsible for organizing programmes in the population groups to which they themselves belonged. Three 'community coordinators' were thus hired in the pilot-phase, one from each of the communities chosen. It had been decided to focus prevention efforts on the large Spanish and Portuguese communities (size of the community as a criterion of priority), as well as on the culturally diverse Turkish community (the challenge being here to cope with significant cultural differences).

A second priority was based on residence status. This was to provide information for refugees and people seeking asylum (as well as for seasonal workers, a specific group not discussed here). Particular attention was devoted to refugees and temporarily resident asylum seekers because the majority originate from countries where HIV prevention is not yet a priority (problem specific data), and their knowledge about the disease, risks of infection and protective measures is frequently insufficient. Moreover, information and prevention work is facilitated since they can be reached fairly readily: they live for prolonged periods in facilities under the auspices of Swiss national and local authorities (organizational data leading to good accessibility).

Members of target groups defined by the Swiss national AIDS prevention strategy and who are also migrants deserve special attention. This applies in particular to staff in certain economic sectors (often young single people working in hotels and catering, construction, farming, hospital staff), young people in educational institutions, women, sex workers and clients, injecting drug users, persons in prison or remand custody, gay and bisexual men as well as behaviourally homosexual men who do not consider themselves gay, and illegal aliens. AIDS prevention programmes (provision of specific information and of material) and, in some cases, counselling and support infrastructure, already exist for many of these groups. An important step was to integrate representatives of migrant groups within existing structures, thus ensuring that their interests are taken into account and that information is disseminated to them. As the second phase of the prevention programme is being developed, increasing attention is being paid to these subgroups, who are often minorities within minorities.

Description of the Programme

The very first concern of the national coordinator in charge of the programme for 'AIDS and migrants/ethnic minorities' was to define a clear and efficient prevention strategy. The programme has been developed in collaboration with the countries of origin (becoming aware of the nature of the AIDS campaigns and the epidemiological situation, coordination with health authorities, exchange of information and material, using the media and its extensions in Switzerland, collaboration with authorities in charge of the Diaspora such as the Spanish Emigration Council, and recourse to diplomatic channels).

In accord with the national AIDS prevention strategy, the programme began with raising awareness in target communities in Switzerland. Programme personnel are of the nationalities of the target communities. They have worked in close collaboration with representatives from their countries in the host country, including diplomatic institutions and advisors such as those for education and social affairs; target community delegates at the 'Swiss Federal Commission for Foreign Nationals'; community leaders in charge of a range of organizations such as cultural associations, training programmes, political groups, sports associations, trade unions, social and religious groups, parent–teacher associations and youth associations; media in their language in Switzerland; and 'mediators' and peer educators recruited and trained from each of these levels. Finally, an effort has been made to involve and sensitize Swiss institutions such as national and local authorities concerned

with migration issues, health, asylum seekers and refugees, educational assistance to migrants and ethnic minorities, as well as the Swiss AIDS Foundation,
family planning centres, employment offices, trade unions and professional
organizations, welfare organizations, medical bodies and the media.

Within each of the communities the campaign for raising AIDS awareness was based on the principles that:

1 messages and measures must be adapted to the cultural characteristics of the particular ethnic groups involved;
2 information and motivation activities focusing on self-help and peer-
   education should be promoted and supported;
3 existing structures and channels of information are to be used and
   built upon; and
4 any form of stigmatization of an 'immigrant risk group' is to be
   avoided.

Work with Communities from Traditional Guest-worker Countries

Concrete AIDS prevention measures aimed at the general population of the
three pilot communities, the Spanish, Portuguese and Turkish, began with
provision of information and coordination between all bodies representing
the communities in Switzerland, including embassies, consulates, the Federal
Commission for Foreigners, umbrella and other important organizations,
religious dignitaries, sport clubs, cultural centres, etc. Written information
was sent to all representatives, announcing the beginning of the programme,
and explaining why such a programme had been implemented for migrants
and ethnic minorities.

For the Spanish and Portuguese communities, emphasis was given to
AIDS prevention information sessions organized through a well established
network of associations. A letter presenting the project was sent to at least
600 Spanish and Portuguese associations, along with a questionnaire inquir-
ing about AIDS prevention activities they might already have carried out.
The letter also solicited proposals for establishing a calendar of possible
interventions. Although only few replies were received, the letters served to
inform the organizations of the project's existence, and facilitated future
contact. We later found that previous formal contacts with certain authorities
and officials such as embassies and umbrella organizations were very useful
in providing a 'community agreement' when other organizations asked their
authorities about the project.

In the Turkish community, on the other hand, the network of associations is less developed than in the Spanish and the Portuguese, since
immigration is a relatively recent phenomenon. For this reason, less emphasis
was placed on institutions and more was put on training key informants as

disseminators of AIDS prevention messages and materials. During the initial phase of making contact with the Turkish community, information was gathered about informal channels of communication, and about people who would be trusted and reliable sources of information within the community. Football trainers and religious leaders (Imams) were identified. Training courses were therefore organized for both groups. Thirty football coaches participated in a seminar entitled 'Sport, Health and AIDS', organized in collaboration with the Swiss Football Federation and the Turkish Embassy. All of the seventeen 'official' Imams from throughout Switzerland attended a first AIDS information session for religious leaders, 'Islam and AIDS', in 1992, and during the 1993 Ramadan, AIDS was mentioned in every mosque in Switzerland.

It was felt to be important for the policy maker to encourage religious leaders to talk about the potential danger of AIDS while at the same time respecting their ways of discussing the issue in the context of the laws of Islam, particularly concerning fidelity or methods of protection. An Imam, as a respected religious authority, will be listened to when he speaks about AIDS. Even if his message does not always coincide with the point of view of public health, it can contribute to making his people aware, whilst leaving them the ultimate choice as to the protective behaviour they consider the most suitable.

Workplace interventions to enhance AIDS awareness have been organized with trade unions, employers' associations, etc. in sectors which employ predominantly non-Swiss labour. Avoiding any sign of stigmatization, material is made available to workers in their mother tongue. Distribution of 'reminder' material at strategic information points (e.g. posters about modes of HIV transmission, and reminding that there is virtually no risk of infection at work), appears to be an effective aid to prevention. Training courses for middle management (those with interface functions), conducted in collaboration with the trade unions, are also a suitable platform for the promotion of awareness.

Information channels specifically targeted at the communities have been used for distributing and conveying information, with existing networks being reinforced and extended. Such channels include Spanish, Portuguese and Turkish language radio and television broadcasts on the subject of AIDS, and articles in newspapers and publications by associations and trade unions. The Federal Commission for Foreigners also plays an important political role in displaying information.

Another priority has been to promote training of health advisors, key informants and health promoters from within each of the communities, recruited from medical and paramedical professions as well as among non-professionals in close contact with, and well accepted within, specific groups. At the beginning it was thought to be important that such people possess good knowledge of a Swiss national language so that they could be integrated into already existing training structures. In 1992, a mainstream service in charge of training for AIDS prevention in the French-speaking part of Switzerland organized seminars for liaison workers in the groups covered by the project. A permanent training module for liaison workers from migrant communities and Swiss personnel was subsequently established. We have had to face the fact, however, that a number of key workers, mostly non-professionals, have little knowledge of the official Swiss languages.

Existing school structures (mother-tongue language and culture classes for children, integration classes in Swiss schools, schools for adult education) have been used to organize information and awareness programmes, working through consultative commissions for parents, school councils and departments of education, and teachers. Special attention is paid to second-generation immigrants, who cope with the conflicts of moving between two cultures: brought up according to traditional patterns in the family, they often confront more liberal local customs and patterns of behaviour at school and at work.

Much work has taken place through diplomatic channels, for example through the Emigration Council in Spain which, at the request of national representatives based in Switzerland, encouraged the embassy and consulates to support the programme. The education attaché of the Portuguese embassy is lending official support as teachers of Portuguese language and culture are trained and provided with teaching resources for AIDS prevention. Activity involving national authorities of the country of origin in the process often leads to better involvement of targeted groups, especially when working inside the school system.

Finally, telephone hotlines in several foreign languages function each week throughout the country, some with the cooperation of regional AIDS associations. These hotlines provide personal information and counselling, and offer the opportunity of making an appointment for a personal interview (Burgi, 1995).

Other population groups have been integrated in the prevention programme since 1993. Among them are: Latin-Americans, for whom an entire programme of interventions has taken place; Africans with whom only a few activities have been conducted (especially with asylum seekers); and Arabs for whom an AIDS hotline and information sessions were available for two years. A new pre-programme is being implemented to assess needs and possible response to prevention activities among the Tamil community. One of the core programme staff members is in charge of coordinating activities among such smaller communities, with the help of 'promoters' who speak the languages of these communities.

Information and Prevention among Refugees and Asylum Seekers

Asylum seekers and refugees suffer from a substantial lack of integration and possibilities for networking within Swiss society. For this reason, responsibility for AIDS education falls on the institutions and groups committed to helping them. A comprehensive programme had to involve all responsible bodies at various levels: national, cantonal and local. Establishment of a working group had been planned, made up of representatives of concerned organizations, to determine needs and existing levels of knowledge, and to adapt an information strategy accordingly. Federal authorities in charge of refugees and asylum seekers should have assumed responsibility for this working group. It soon became clear, however, that no concrete measures could be implemented at this level, due especially to administrative complications and unclear definition of responsibilities.

With the support of the Federal Office of Public Health, a pilot project was, however, developed at the cantonal level in Geneva to address issues of HIV prevention among refugees and asylum seekers. Involving local government and non-government organizations in charge of asylum seekers and refugees, the aim of the project was to train staff members and nurses working in asylum seekers' residence centres how to conduct a culturally adapted prevention session. The project also involves asylum seekers as peer-educators, who have developed a multicultural theatre play. It has been monitored continuously (Haour-Knipe *et al.*, 1995), and is intended to serve as a model for other cantons. The play has now been recorded on video-tape, guidelines established for asylum seekers ('how to inform my friends and colleagues within the community'), and recommendations formulated for staff members and counsellors on organizing AIDS prevention sessions (Chaignat *et al.*, 1995). These are to be distributed to the major local authorities and non-government organizations. Workshops, training, and information sessions are planned for local government authorities, social workers and nurses in the centres themselves.

At the same time, AIDS information booklets are distributed within preliminary reception centres under federal responsibility during the first days after an asylum seekers' arrival in Switzerland. Posters inform asylum seekers that they can receive free condoms 'protecting against unwanted pregnancy, AIDS, and other sexually transmitted diseases' while they are confined in centres at the border. Since local AIDS units are very often perceived as 'the specialists' for AIDS prevention, special training sessions are offered for their personal, informing them about the pilot-project for asylum seekers. Participants are taught how to use the material available, and what methods they could use to inform asylum seekers and refugees when asked to do so by local authorities or NGOs.

Non-nationals as Subgroups of other Target Groups

While efforts towards the general population (information sessions, production of adapted materials, involvement of community-based media, workplace and school interventions) have been maintained, from 1994 onwards greater emphasis has been placed on involving specific target groups and key personnel within them during a second phase of the programme. Targeted activities have involved adolescents, illegal aliens, women, injecting drug users, and behaviourally homosexual men (with or without 'gay' identity). Since prevention programmes for specific target groups already exist, the main concern here has been to integrate migrants and ethnic minorities' issues into these programmes.

In practice, we have found it difficult to integrate the specific problems of migrant populations here: the more precisely the programme needs to be targeted, the more it involves specialized organizations (gays, women, or those active in the field of drug dependence). These seldom have experience working with those who are not Swiss, and very few successfully make the link with migrant communities. Furthermore, professionals active in these fields very rarely have immigrant backgrounds themselves. If specialized organizations are occasionally aware of the specific needs of migrants and ethnic minorities, they do not know how to include them in their plans of action, or are simply unable to reach these communities.

Our strategy has thus been one of infiltration. We have provided skills and developed specific 'community-based subgroup projects' aimed at migrant adolescents, women, injecting drug users, gay and behaviourally homosexual men. Once these projects, carried out by trained volunteers, are under way and made known to the communities or to the people concerned, the idea is to gradually integrate them into mainstream services or existing programmes through official requests for support. Both the promotion of the institutional capacities of the migrants involved in a project (their problem-specific knowledge and learning 'how to sell an existing project to a Swiss organization') and the inclination of the local institutions to include non-national into their activities are at stake. The idea is to generate a dynamic process originating in the communities. The process is facilitated if examples of ongoing projects are available to Swiss organizations, along with identified representatives of the migrant communities.

Finally, the idea of promoting multicultural projects within existing institutional frameworks must be pursued. A suitable and feasible project which includes several communities stands better chances of succeeding. Up to now, at least in Switzerland, it would have been unrealistic to request that public health authorities and organizations take into account each of many cultural and ethnic particularities or nuances in their approaches. To include persons from the communities at all steps of the development of a specific programme fosters better understanding of these issues. Three examples of prevention work among some of these subgroups, clandestine migrants, young people, and men who have sex with men, are presented below:

An Outreach Project Aimed at Latin-American Women Working as (often Illegal) Child-Minders

People living illegally in Switzerland seldom contact health and/or social services since they are afraid to become known to local authorities. Many women without legal status mind children, and a strategy was developed to reach these people where they are. Most of the women are very young, and come from countries where AIDS information and prevention might not be optimal (Ospina and Burgi, 1995).

In Geneva many such women from Latin-America meet during the summer in city and suburban parks with the children for whom they are caring, so four project workers from different Latin-American countries were identified and trained to talk with them. The main print support for this approach was a free comic book with a colourful, but non-explicit, cover and a story about AIDS, which women could read while the children were playing. Project workers held short or in-depth discussions with about 600 women in eleven parks (two visits per week in each park during the summer). Only seven were not interested in receiving information. Sixteen per cent of the women spontaneously sought contact a second or third time. Most had specific questions after the first contact, or after reading the comic book. The women contacted were invited to a monthly meeting in a place which had no explicit link with AIDS, where further discussions could be held about topics of interest to them, including legal issues. Attendance at the monthly meeting was low, but some women mentioned that, although hesitant to come due to their illegal status, they had done so because the facilitators were women who had themselves been in the same situation.

Spanish Youth Theatre Project

Young Spanish people living in Switzerland are quite well informed about HIV and AIDS, but may have difficulties discussing these topics within their families. They may not, for example, know the 'right words' in their mother tongue to use with their parents. There may be conflict between generations about such things as the way to experience sexuality, or male and female roles in relationships. The aim of the youth theatre project was to point out the most frequent obstacles to condom use, to provide information in a humorous way, to discuss the attitudes of women and to stimulate their preventive behaviour, as well as to train the young people involved in conveying HIV prevention messages (Cristobal, 1993).

The actors are 'second generation' Spanish young people, members of a Spanish Youth association in Lucerne. The idea of staging a play emerged in the association after an information event about AIDS. With the help of two adults, the young people wrote a script based on a Swiss story. They modified the text to reflect the language and expressions of Spanish immigrants. The play stimulated a great deal of discussion: it aroused inhibitions and resistance among the actors, and audiences perceived a discrepancy between their female/male roles in the play and in real life. All these aspects were discussed after the performances, with the participation of the actors. The play has been performed sixteen times throughout the country, mostly for Spanish associations, trade unions, and schools, and has reached about 1 200 spectators. The actors have been trained as mediators/peer educators. They have since developed a new play on drug issues, focusing on misunderstandings, on communication problems and on social difficulties within and outside the family. This play is now being performed in different Swiss cities within the Spanish network, with the support of a Swiss organization dealing with drugs and health-promotion issues.

Work among Spanish Men Who Have Sex with Men in Switzerland

A number of Spaniards living with HIV or AIDS in Switzerland are gay. When confronted with illness or after taking risks, some call the Spanish AIDS hotline: only a few benefit from minimal support networks. Whether or not they socialize with the homosexual milieu, some live out their homosexuality quite openly. A considerable proportion have left families and friends in Spain in order to do so, away from social constraints. If they become infected or ill, their already precarious situation in relation to the employment or studies which permit their status as residents in Switzerland is endangered. They may feel very lonely, without effective social or family support. Other Spaniards, born in Switzerland, often from modest and rather traditional origins, do not dare come out to peers as gay. They feel burdened by a certain kind of social control, and tend to avoid the Swiss gay community. Some have gathered around the first Spanish lesbian and gay association in Switzerland.

The policy maker's task in this instance consists of a multilevel intervention, working both with local and with migrant gay groups. Programme workers have, for example, encouraged Swiss gay associations to try to integrate migrant gay organizations into their information and prevention networks, and to become aware of the situation of such people as the 'Portuguese friend', who may have been met last summer in his home country and brought to Switzerland for the sake of a relationship. Local organizations of people with AIDS, and non-government organizations active in prevention, are encouraged to identify the specific needs of HIV infected gay migrants (whether or not they define themselves as gay) and to help professionals from specialized services find adequate answers to their counselling and support needs. Within the Spanish community, the taboo surrounding homosexuality is being fought by letting gay people express their views in preventive material and activities, and by emphasizing solidarity and non-discrimination. This method is also being applied with injecting drug users.

'Mediators' as Peer-educators

AIDS prevention activities with the various migrant populations living in Switzerland could not have been conducted in such range and depth without the contribution of the approximately 120 'mediators and multipliers', professionals and non-professionals from the Spanish, Portuguese, Turkish and other communities. Those who were to become mediators made themselves known during prevention activities for the general population, as well in the course of specific projects for target groups (youth, drug users, gays, women, etc.). Some spontaneously offered to help organize prevention activities, while others helped to facilitate the programme's activities from within key positions in schools, unions, umbrella organizations for migrants, the media and so forth. All belong to the population groups at which the programmes are aimed.

Several kinds of training have been offered. Some mediators were simply trained on the spot, while working in the community with the coordinator. Others have requested special training, of which three options have been made available:

1. specific training on AIDS and prevention within the project for the collaborators of a given community (open to all, or in specialized groups such as teachers or football coaches);
2. formal training on AIDS prevention in different cultures, a course given within the framework of a national general AIDS training programme (available to both migrant collaborators and Swiss professionals or volunteers working with migrant communities); and
3. global training with non-government organizations specialized in prevention and health promotion within migrant communities, as discussed in the example below.

In addition, numerous single events such as seminars or conferences have been held to enhance awareness among Swiss prevention workers, especially local public health authorities and heads of support or health organizations.

Living with One's Peers: An Example of Health Promotion at 'Appartenances'

Appartenances, in French, implies 'belonging'. Misfortune acts as a separator, and AIDS separates us from others, forcing us into new networks, such as those to do with health care. Individuals struggle to remain attached, however, searching for solutions with the help of close friends and family. It is in this way that individuals become innovators, becoming authors of their own future rather than prey or victims of fate. Such a process may mean going through a period of being misunderstood by others, or of estrangement from the norms of the society in which they are living. This is especially so in the case of immigrant communities, who are often already excluded, but who are nonetheless innovators and producers of new forms of society.

To realize the idea of global, active community health prevention, the Appartenances Association in the city of Lausanne decided to organize training of promoters, persons from immigrant communities interested in working with people in need within their own communities, on the individual, familial or community level. Such a programme is only possible with the help of contact persons, or multipliers, professionals and non-professionals in contact with local organizations and networks, whether monocultural or multicultural. These contact persons train the promoters, directly in prevention of HIV or indirectly in relation to other types of exclusion. This prevention work entails the concerns of health professionals involved in the fight against AIDS in migrant communities living in Switzerland, but originally evolved from field experience in developing countries (Métraux and Aviles, 1992; Métraux and Fleury, 1995; Métraux, Mihoubi and Brogli, 1995) where there may be few professionals, and especially where programmes imposed from above, which fail to take into account the communities concerned, have failed, and where community involvement is thus indispensable.

Training begins by establishing the needs of each group of participants through a community diagnosis. This diagnosis often reveals lack of information, inaccessibility to institutions and to power in the host country, and difficulties in changing individual behaviour and habits in the face of social controls from one's own culture. Training uses the themes developed through this first analysis. In a first phase, individual experience is explored, the emotional experience at the time of an important change in a participant's life, along with the solutions, hindrances, resources and defences discovered in overcoming the crisis. The next phase, that of belonging to the group, allows for the elaboration of guidelines of transcultural invariables which form the basis for elaborating teaching material or community tools. The third phase is one of experience with the knowledge acquired during the training. This usually takes place in the form of role-playing. Role-playing allows the participant to bring back into the present that which, in its absence, has often became a fixation or source of disturbance. Identifying

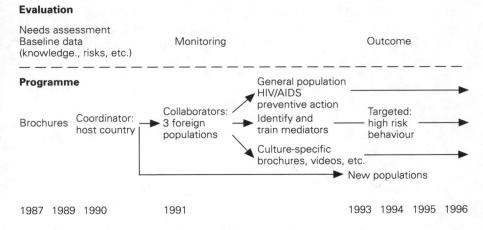

Figure 9.2 AIDS prevention programme for migrants and ethnic minorities in Switzerland

needs is the door by which contact is made with the members of the promoter's group.

Summary and Prospects

The AIDS prevention programme for migrants and ethnic minorities in Switzerland can be summarized schematically as in Figure 9.2.

Accompanied by ongoing evaluation (baseline, monitoring, and impact), the programme has defined specific targets, for example: 'By the end of 1996, immigrant community educators should have been recruited and trained, particularly in the context of such specific target groups as women, homosexuals, and sex workers' or 'By the end of 1998, 90 per cent of the immigrant population should have been reached by AIDS prevention measures that take into account their ethnic and cultural characteristics'. The programme is based on a principle of reaching people through the use of ever-expanding networks: a Swiss coordinator was joined by collaborators from each of the communities chosen for the pilot phase, who in turn have identified and trained more than 120 'mediators' in their respective communities (Burgi *et al.*, 1994; Burgi *et al.*, 1996).

Work in the immediate future is taking two new directions: towards additional migrant communities, and towards other prevention activities. Two additional 'national coordinators' have recently joined the staff, one Italian and the other originating in the Kosovo district of the former Yugoslavia. In summer 1995, the national 'Migrants and AIDS prevention project' officially became the 'Migrants and health promotion project'. Based on the same principles, the programme will now include other health promotion and prevention issues under federal responsibility, such as those of legal and illegal drugs. The new direction reflects the practical difficulty experienced in fieldwork of including both general and specific populations, such as women or youth, in a strategy narrowed to one single theme, often taboo, such as AIDS. Health promotion, in fact, avoids fragmentation into precise yet restricted themes. More importantly, it is impossible to prevent diseases without paying attention to the overall well-being of migrant communities.

References

BURGI, D. (1991) 'AuslanderInnen in der Schweiz: Eine andere Sprache und ein unterschiedlicher Ansatz bei der AIDS-Prävention', in *Mäglichkeiten und Grenzen der Präventionsstrategien im Gesundheitsbereich am Beispiel AIDS*, Begleitbroschure zum Symposium des Bundesamtes für Gesundheitswesen, Berne, October 1991.

BURGI, D. (1995) 'Analyse des appels parvenus aux permanences téléphoniques en langues étrangères concernant le Sida', Université de Lausanne: Institut de Psychologie.

BURGI, D., CARVALHO, E., CRISTOBAL, M., DEMIRKAN, H., OSPINA, S. and CARRON R. (1996) 'Projet migrants: Rapport d'activités 1993–5, Prévention du Sida auprès des communautés espagnoles, portugaises, turques et latino-américaines en Suisse', Berne: Office Fédéral de la Santé Publique.

BURGI, D., CRISTOBAL, M., DEMIRKAN, H. and OSPINA, S. (1994) 'Projet migrants: Rapport final 1991/92', Berne: Office Fédéral de la Santé Publique.

CHAIGNAT, C.-L., OSPINA, S., HAOUR-KNIPE, M., FLEURY, F., LUCKE, A. and LOUTAN, L. (1995) 'Prévention du Sida chez les requérants d'asile à Genève: Rapport final du projet pilote' Genève; Unité de Médecine Communautaire, Hôpital Cantonal Universitaire.

CRISTOBAL, M. (1993) 'AIDS prevention: Performance of the AIDS Group of young People of the Lucerne Theatre', in DEUTSCH AIDS-HILFE (Ed.) *Migrants, Ethnic Minorities and AIDS: First European Meeting for the Exchange of Information*, pp. 53–4, Blossin, May.

DUBOIS-ARBER, F., LEHMANN, P., HAUSSER, D. and GUTZWILER, F. (1989) *Evaluation des Campagnes de Prévention du Sida en Suisse: Deuxième Rapport de Synthèse, 1988*, Lausanne: IUMSP Doc. 39.

FLEURY, F. (1989) *Evaluation des Campagnes de Prévention du Sida en Suisse: Les Migrants, Rapport Final, 1988*, Lausanne: IUMSP Doc. 39.5.

FLEURY, F. (1990) 'Sida/migration/prévention. Dossier turc' (unpublished).

FLEURY, F. (1991) 'Swiss report', in HAOUR-KNIPE, M. *Assessing AIDS Prevention: Migrants and Travellers Group Final Report*, Lausanne: IUMSP Doc. 72.

FLEURY, F. and HAOUR-KNIPE, M. (1993) *Sida/Migration/Prévention, Projet Migrants: Monitoring 1992–3*, Lausanne: IUMSP Doc. 82.7.

FLEURY, F., HAOUR-KNIPE, M. and OSPINA, S. (1991) *Sida/Migration/Prévention: Dossier Portugais, Dossier Espagnol, 1989–90,* Lausanne: IUMSP Doc. 52.7.

HAOUR-KNIPE, M., OSPINA, S., FLEURY, F., CHAIGNAT, C.-L., LUCKE, A. and LOUTAN, L. (1995) 'Evaluation of an HIV/AIDS prevention programme: Newly-arrived asylum seekers', *AIDS in Europe: The Behavioural Aspect, Vol. 4,* pp. 191–8, Berlin: Editions Sigma.

HAOUR-KNIPE, M., OSPINA, S., FLEURY, F., JEANGROS, C. and DUBOIS-ARBER, F. (1993) 'Evaluation des connaissances et comportements relatifs au Sida des travailleurs saisonniers en Suisse', *Médecine Sociale et Préventive,* **38,** pp. 58–63.

HAOUR-KNIPE, M., OSPINA, S., FLEURY, F. and ZIMMERMANN, E. (1992) 'HIV/AIDS knowledge and migrant workers', in AGGLETON, P., HART, G. and DAVIES, P. (Eds) *AIDS: Rights, Risk and Reason,* pp. 85–101, London: Falmer Press.

MÉTRAUX, J.-C. and AVILES, A. (1992) 'Training techniques for non-professionals: A Nicaraguan preventive and primary care mental health programme', in McCULLIN, M. (Ed.) *The Psychological Well Being of Refugee Children: Research, Practice and Policy Issues,* pp. 226–43, Geneva: International Catholic Child Bureau.

MÉTRAUX, J.-C. and FLEURY, F. (1995) 'Creators of their future: Group work with traumatized communities', in PERREN, G. (Ed.) *Trauma, Culture and Emotion: The Healing Power of Groups,* Bern: Paul Verlag.

MÉTRAUX, J.-C., MIHOUBI, S. and BROGLI, N. (1995) 'Entraide et exclusion', *Revue Médicale de la Suisse Romande,* **115,** pp. 481–3.

OSPINA, S. and BURGI, D. (1995) 'An AIDS prevention strategy for a recently arrived and unstructured migrant population, Latin Americans in Switzerland', *AIDS in Europe: The Behavioural Aspects, Vol. 3,* pp. 135–8, Berlin: Editions Sigma.

OSPINA, S., CRISTOBAL, M., DEMIRKAN, H. and BURGI, D. (1993) 'AIDS prevention: Reaching the immigrant population in Switzerland', in DEUTSCH AIDS-HILFE (Ed.) *Migrants, Ethnic Minorities and AIDS: First European Meeting for the Exchange of Information,* pp. 50–3, Blossin, May.

Chapter 10

Care Issues and Migrants

Maureen Louhenapessy

The Universal Declaration of The Rights of AIDS and HIV Patients, drawn up by *Aides* and *Médecins du Monde*, states: persons infected with the virus are protected by common law. No special legislation may apply to them (para. 2); persons infected with the virus must have unrestricted access to care (para. 3); the freedom or rights of persons shall not be restricted for the sole reason that they are infected with the virus, whatever their race, nationality, religion, sex or sexual orientation (para. 5); and under no circumstances may an individual be screened for the virus without his knowledge (para. 8).

This declaration was drawn up in 1987. Ten years later we are forced to conclude that there have been many infringements, from an ethical, human, racial and social point of view. Many recommendations have been made at local, national and international levels against the targeting of a particular population, calling for living and socio-economic conditions to be taken into account, and demanding that care for AIDS patients should not be seen in isolation from preventive measures. Despite all these recommendations, we have continued to fail to meet our objectives, and to organize prevention strategies which ultimately prove counter-productive.

We have had to fight against society's instinctive fear of an epidemic which comes from elsewhere and which is brought by somebody else — by the 'foreigner'. The foreigner provides a prime, ready-made target. In Belgium, it is the African community in general, and the Zairian community in particular, which have been singled out in this way. Bideau (1991) writes in his article 'Africa, the imaginary land of AIDS':

> Many articles published by leading scientific journals continue to trundle out the same old clichés and stereotypes . . . to invent an Africa which probably only exists in the imagination of Western scholars themselves. Not only are the ethnographic facts often biased, false or unverifiable, they are also placed in an inadequate interpretative context . . .

[He also quotes from Mudimbe's very beautiful book *The Invention of Africa*]
More than anything else, the traditional depiction of Africa by Westerners shows us how they generally project their fantasies onto a dark, savage and primitive continent, where attitudes and behaviour are imagined to be the opposite of what is found in the west.

All these fears and clichés have led migrant populations, feeling 'accused' or 'stigmatized', to shut themselves off from the prevention process, and reinforced a refusal to accept the reality of AIDS. Feelings of guilt are reinforced for persons living with HIV, driving them into an anonymous existence on the fringes of society. It is a considerable challenge to implement prevention and psycho-social support programmes for migrant populations in such a context. In implementing specific programmes, we must be careful not to further marginalize and to stigmatize, but rather to clearly target and define measures in such a way that they can be understood and accepted by migrants. In 1985, we thus decided to develop culturally and linguistically appropriate prevention programmes which directly involve both the communities and the organizations in direct contact with them.

Approach to the Situation in Belgium

To properly understand the choices made in the field of prevention in Belgium, it is important to present the situation as a whole. We have been faced with the problem of AIDS in migrant communities since the very start of the epidemic. As early as 1981, hospitals were treating patients from Zaire, Rwanda and Burundi, former colonies with historic links to Belgium. In 1985 we established our first information programme, and by 1986 the project was well and truly under way. From the very beginning we organized prevention strategies which included social support for people living with HIV and AIDS. We will now look at how administrative, legal and social problems are inextricably linked to the cultural approach.

HIV Testing

Although HIV testing in Belgium is voluntary, discriminatory measures have been taken against certain persons. Students requesting a grant from the Agence Gouvernemetale de Coopération au Développement (AGCD), for example, are required to submit a certificate confirming that they have been tested negative for HIV. The testing takes place in the country of origin, and a seropositive result prevents the student from coming to Belgium. Testing on entry into Belgium principally concerns asylum seekers. The measures range from systematic screening to no testing at all. The result, a state of confusion and discriminatory decisions, has a negative effect on the scope for prevention among the migrant populations. Migrants lose confidence in the Belgian system of health care, and are afraid that an HIV-positive status will be used as grounds for refusing to grant them a residence permit in Belgium. This fear leads certain individuals to drop out of the social and medical circuit altogether — only to reappear when they actually become ill with AIDS.

Administrative and Ethical Problems

After arriving in Belgium and requesting political asylum, individuals are either housed in Red Cross reception centres or register with the Centre Public d'Aide Sociale (CPAS) in the commune in which they reside. In either case, they are entitled to receive a document known as a *réquisitoire médical* which covers medical expenses. Some CPAS offices fail to grant this document to persons who are nevertheless legally entitled to one. There are 95 per cent of asylum requests which are refused by the Office des Etrangers (Aliens Office). Asylum seekers may appeal against this decision, pending which they are entitled to social and medical assistance. Many people do not receive such assistance, however, and we are obliged to exert pressure on the CPAS offices in order to ensure that they respect the ban. During the period pending appeal, we often have to ask charity organizations such as Exil or Médecins Sans Frontières to provide medical treatment for asylum seekers, and since they do not have a sufficient infrastructure for the most serious cases, some individuals are ultimately cared for by hospital emergency services. The health of these individuals can be compromised by these administrative irregularities, the lack of access to housing, the cessation of medication, the absence of blood tests, and the unavailability of AZT.

Rejected asylum seekers may request an extension of their stay in Belgium for medical reasons, but there is no legislation governing such a procedure, and it remains a purely administrative decision, taken by an official at the *Office des Etrangers*. The request for an extended stay for medical reasons is made on humanitarian grounds. A kind of 'blackmail' operates at present: if case workers say from what disease the patient is suffering, then he or she may be granted an extended stay, but this practice is generally unacceptable to the patient, the medical profession and social workers. It is contrary to all accepted ethics.

The status of sick children is linked to that of their parents, but their medical condition is taken into account when deciding to grant a possible extension to the parents. If they are orphaned, their residence rights become a very complicated matter, with many administrative obstacles. The most significant obstacle is the request by the Belgian authorities for a legal birth certificate. As many asylum seekers come from countries which are at war or in administrative turmoil following looting, such as Zaire, this requirement poses enormous problems. All of these administrative procedures have an effect on migrants living with HIV and AIDS, and serve to push them to the fringes of society or even exclude them altogether. In such circumstances, how can we speak of proper patient care and access to treatment?

Why Develop Specific Programmes?

For the past thirty-five years, the *Service Social des Etrangers* has been an institution devoted to implementing actions targeted primarily at the under-privileged. It attaches particular importance to setting up programmes adapted to migrants and refugees who face integration problems. Over the years, the *Service Social des Etrangers* has developed a solid infrastructure consisting of nine centres running polyvalent social action projects (social, cultural and occupational integration). Its concern has been to develop programmes which respect individuals and cultures, to combat all forms of discrimination, and to prevent marginalization and exclusion. The fight against HIV transmission has now been part of this process for almost ten years.

The *Service Social des Etrangers* is also responsible for coordinating and implementing primary preventive measures targeted specifically at migrant populations. The latter are identified as a target group on the basis of characteristics such as language difficulties, cultural perceptions, social and legal barriers, socio-economic status which is often unfavourable, internal social organization, religion, vulnerability linked to refugee status, and mobility. All these factors directly influence the impact of general programmes on the migrant population. They also have an impact on the care and support for people living with AIDS and HIV.

The migrant population is heterogeneous — as is the population as a whole. Groups and subgroups differ as to geographical origin, the period of immigration, reasons for residence in Belgium, level of education, employment and income, recent arrival as a political refugee, and experiences in the country of origin. All these parameters influence the approach that must be adopted in order to ensure that preventive measures actually work. Activities are designed for or meet the needs and priorities of so-called 'vulnerable' groups. These groups experience both socio-economic and cultural difficulties which affect their access to information, acceptance of information, and attitudes concerning health problems. All these factors apply to the AIDS issue, a situation in fact made even more problematic by the cultural pressure and social control exercised within certain groups.

The programmes developed directly involve the communities in the prevention process at the grass-roots level, allowing us to combat denial and ignorance more effectively, and ensuring that they take account of the real needs of the population. Social and legal support for people living with HIV and AIDS is an inherent part of the prevention process. Socio-economic status which is often fragile, and lack of housing, or dependency on temporary accommodation with friends or family, means that people may move around frequently, and are without a fixed address. In this case, the *Service Social des Etrangers* social network may be the only institution able to help them, in circumstances which, moreover, often exclude the patient from any health-care system. The first step is to prevent any further marginalization, by ensuring that every individual has access to available care and support (physiotherapy, psychological counselling, etc.). By organizing adequate legal support, we are able to ensure that many people who would otherwise be excluded are able to gain access to the health-care system.

The Health Model

State-provided health services in Europe tend to be based on a highly specialized and technological model. In other parts of the world, health models are still strongly influenced by culture and tradition. The first point of contact for health care may not necessarily be the general practitioner or the hospital; traditional care or practices used in the family are often the first resort. If a doctor has already made a diagnosis, this must often be confirmed or discredited 'by the tradition' or by an individual who embodies this tradition. The family and the community also play a major role in the recognition and acceptance of illness. Most of the immigrant communities with which we work also use traditional forms of medicine. This must be borne in mind when providing support for patients who may not always be able to situate themselves in relation to western models.

Culturally Appropriate Approaches

When we speak of AIDS, we immediately come up against cultural sensibilities. AIDS inevitably involves discussion of such subjects as sexuality, relationships, women's roles, illness, hospitalization, blood, death, mourning, the illness of a child, etc. Each individual will experience these issues according to his or her own sensibility, culture and living conditions in the host country. The vulnerability of some people may be such that their health has ceased to be a priority concern; there may be more urgent needs to sort out, such as problems with a residence permit, or finding housing or a means of subsistence. Taking all these elements into account, it is important for field workers to understand the different ways in which people look upon illness in general and AIDS in particular. This can be the basis for a better 'communication'. Many care-givers complain of the patient's 'silence', lack of interest in preventive measures, difficulty speaking about the result of an HIV test, or using condoms. The health need of migrants must be seen in a broad context. If communications strategies are to be effective, they must be developed in line with the cultural traditions of individuals. The socioeconomic and socio-political context in which groups are living in the host country must be taken into account when seeking to convey essential messages. The approach to different groups must be progressive in order to overcome cultural barriers.

In overcoming communication problems, particularly difficult when it comes to health, the first rule is to show an interest in the other person, as it is that individual who possesses the information concerning his or her real needs. Each person has his or her own conception of their health and of how to conserve it. But how are we to be sensitive to another person's culture and traditions? We will now attempt to identify a number of elements which may be involved when providing support for a migrant person while taking these cultural factors into account. We will take actual cases as our basis. We should also point out that the communities we work with are mainly of Central African origin (Zaire, Rwanda and Burundi) and Morocco. We also stress that many of those with whom our work takes place have received only limited education, a factor very directly influencing the nature of the approach adopted. This level of education influences the migrant's understanding of health matters and their readiness to accept interventions. Some examples of the everyday reasoning encountered include responses such as: 'How can you be contagious if you are not actually ill?'; 'A good doctor should be able to know immediately whether blood is healthy or not, a doctor who has to keep taking tests can't be very capable'; and 'How can a disease in the blood be sexually transmitted?' These differences in understanding, linked to poor knowledge of how the body works and, on occasion, cultural beliefs such as those regarding the possible mixing of body liquids (sperm and mother's milk, for example), make it difficult to integrate notions of a virus that causes AIDS, its method of transmission and its action on the immune system.

Customary Forms of Greeting

Every culture has its own forms of greeting which are very important, determining the way the conversation will develop. Many patients do not understand the 'cold' and unwelcoming way in which they are greeted by some carers. On the other hand, many carers complain of the 'silence' of patients. Greetings often contain questions and information about health, the family, the children, etc. It may also be customary to wish someone good health and a safe journey when you part. Greetings are also an expression of interest in the other person and can lead to the beginning of a process of communication between two people. Health is generally an important element in these greetings.

Discovering One's Illness

In the societies of origin of our patients, illness is often seen as being caused by elements independent of the individual, the work of spirits, the curse of ancestors, a jinx, the evil eye. The solution to the problem therefore lies with the individuals who are able to understand such things: the shaman, the sorcerer, the marabout, the fetishist.

> Mr A, a Zairian, comes to see us after having received his test results. He has been told he is HIV positive. He is unable to grasp the situation, is totally shattered and keeps asking 'who?' Who has got it in for him, who has brought this 'evil' upon him? He is angry at the hospital, and the carer keeps asking him about his sexuality, his experiences, his wife who has stayed behind in Zaire. He does not see what all this has to do with his 'problem', does not want to return to Zaire, and does not want to answer questions like this. He says he has just received a letter from his wife saying that his youngest child has died. . . . Mr A has no doubt: somebody has got it in for him, and has put a curse on him. He could not have caught this disease by chance and his child could not have died by chance. He asks for social assistance to buy some telephone cards. There are people back in Zaire he wants to contact so that they can make some inquiries and track down the 'fetishist'. He sends a lot of letters . . . For three months there is no news, but Mr A remains convinced that once he has found the individual responsible all his problems will be solved. He will no longer be ill, and will regain his strength . . . One Thursday morning Mr A turns up. He knows who it is; his sister-in-law, it has been shown to him in a dream. This is how he describes it: 'My blood was strange, dirty and bubbling, my sister-in-law was behind our house, stirring a calabash . . . she had thrown her sister into the pot, my baby and my blood . . . My family are now working for me back home, to protect me and to cure me . . . so that I can regain my strength.

We must take all of this on board, as it will enable us to understand why some people may feel 'detached' from their infection. We believe it is important to give people the chance to express these thoughts: they must be given the time to find 'their response' to the problem, after which they may be more willing to accept the support offered to them by the hospital or other services. Some carers will find it difficult to do this, because they perceive such accounts as 'too irrational'. Additionally, throughout the course of the illness patients may continue to use a healer or marabout. Others will turn to prayer groups (some of which may go as far as to claim that the AIDS is in remission and that the person is cured). We must remain attentive to these practices in order not to place them into diametric opposition to medical and psycho-social support: the patient must also be allowed to combine the two approaches, and not feel obliged to choose between them. We have found that those who feel condemned or misunderstood frequently disappear until hospitalization becomes necessary. We must also remember that people in vulnerable situations (financial, of residence status) are often particularly attracted to such practices, in the belief that no other solutions are open to them.

Close links often need to be maintained with the country of origin in order to find solutions to health problems. In the case of Mr A we also saw how he failed to understand the relevance of questions about his lifestyle, sexuality and relationship with his wife. Discussions of this kind are not entered into, and especially not with a stranger, being seen as 'shameful'. Also, if you keep repeating the word AIDS you may end up 'conjuring up the disease' and attracting the evil eye; the less you mention it the better! In the example we have given, we have seen the importance attached to the interpretation of dreams. In addition to discovering who was responsible for putting a curse on him, Mr A also understood what this illness represented. In his dream he saw 'a bubbling of his blood', and it was in these terms that he conceived his HIV infection and AIDS.

Treatment Offered to People Living with HIV

Mr D tells his social worker:

> Since I have known about my 'problem' I have never felt ill. The doctor prescribed a treatment and now I am feeling worse and worse. He's killing me with his medicine. I don't want to go to this doctor any more. I have had some plants sent from my country, they will be better. They are plants to give me back my strength, to strengthen my blood. I don't trust him any more, he is giving me bad medicine because I am a foreigner.

It is sometimes difficult to understand the nature of 'side effects'. Some patients have little or no command of the host country's language, and do not understand the doctor's explanations. This leads us to the problem of translation. Sometimes patients are accompanied by family members (brothers, sisters, children) or friends to serve as translators. This then poses the problem of confidentiality. There have been instances in which it is only while translating that a family member realizes the patient is infected with the AIDS virus, which obviously comes as a shock. Patients may also place great faith in western medicine and fail to understand what is happening if they do not feel well after taking the drugs prescribed. They may think they are being deliberately given the wrong drugs. It is important to spend sufficient time explaining the side effects that may appear.

There is also the question of the environment in which patients are living. Some may be living in a hostel, reception centre or communal house, and it has sometimes been necessary to oblige people to leave these centres when other tenants fear infection and where the infrastructure does not make it possible to provide the necessary care.

Mr E is holding his head in his hands:

> I am tired. I have just come out of hospital, but because I don't have anywhere to live or any money I am staying with friends. I am afraid of moving in this house, of using the bathroom or the kitchen, because there are children living there and I would not like them to catch anything . . . and anyway they hide the food, they don't want to share it because they can't afford it. I have to eat properly, sleep a lot, and look after myself. But how? My family's arriving in ten days, and I must find another solution. I can't look after myself and I prefer to go to hospital where I would have a roof over my head, proper food and rest.

Mr E died shortly afterwards. He had been taken to hospital by ambulance after he collapsed in the street. This example provides a tragic illustration of just how important it is to take into account the social and financial circumstances of patients. While there have been some dramatic developments in modern medicine, support for patients has become increasingly difficult due to the slowly deteriorating social situation and the lack of funds. Growing administrative difficulties prevent social integration and make access to care increasingly difficult. We often have to call upon the services of *Médecins Sans Frontières* and other organizations to treat patients in extremely precarious situations. Some are hospitalized in order to obtain necessary support: hospitalization that could have been avoided had other solutions been available. The example of Mr E also shows the difficulty of finding assistance within a community where living conditions are often so precarious that mutual assistance has become impossible.

Hospitalization

> Ms C has been hospitalized with pulmonary complications. When we visit her she explains that she has left her eldest daughter (aged fifteen) at home. She asks us to go and see her, so that her daughter can prepare her something to eat. She also asks us to buy her cream for her skin, which is becoming uncomfortably dry in the cold northern climate. She is unable to eat the hospital food and asks us why she is being given water. The contents of her drip look like water . . .

Patients often ask to be given their usual food when they are hospitalized. This may be for religious reasons (Islam, for example) or simply not to change their customary diet. Certain beliefs, moreover, are linked to diet, where certain foods are recommended when one is ill, and certain plants and decoctions for specific complaints. For members of the family, also, it can be very important to continue to prepare food for the patient as a means of continuing to care for them.

As for treatment and medical care, it is very important to explain exactly what is being done and why, to make sure that medical treatment is correctly interpreted.

> Mr B, for example, complained about the frequency of the blood samples:
> If he goes on taking my blood I will grow weaker and weaker; he should give me blood, and not take so much.

Loneliness is a problem for many patients who, when they are hospitalized, have not wished to tell members of their own community about their illness. Since they must therefore overcome many social, financial and other problems without calling on their friends, they may become more dependent on the hospital psycho-social team and on external social services. They are also sometimes faced with some very difficult decisions regarding their children and their future. Some ask to go back to their own country before it is too late.

Home care may be difficult to arrange, partly for financial reasons, but also because accommodation is cramped or inadequate, or because the patient may be sharing with others. In these cases a patient must often therefore remain in hospital. Others find it very difficult to get to the hospital for regular out-patient care, or to go to the chemist with their prescriptions. It is important to be able to make the patient's community aware of all these problems in order to set up a help network within that community, while always bearing in mind that there will be some patients who will never turn to that community for fear that their secret will be 'betrayed'. Some patients are willing to accept help from a voluntary worker; it is therefore important to ensure that these voluntary workers receive training in the cultural approach. Patients often request spiritual help. Sometimes this means someone outside the hospital, and sometimes the services provided by the hospital are sufficient (e.g. via a priest, Protestant chaplain, Imam).

Death: Mourning

Ms K is very ill. It is time to make a decision about a host family for her children since she is very frightened of them being sent back to their home country. She refuses to tell them that she is going to die, though.

> Who can say when you are going to die except God? He alone knows. Nobody here can say when I am going to die . . . There are things I must say and do . . . before. There's my mother back home, I can't go before she does. She still needs me. . . . I must speak to X. He must speak with my family back there.

A discussion of death brings us right to the heart of the complexity of a culturally sensitive approach. 'Only God knows when you are going to die' is a widely held belief, and makes discussion with the families and the patient very difficult. In this case the support team did not manage to convince the patient to talk to her children and prepare them for her death.

There are also certain customary rites for some migrant groups, such as 'being heard before you die' so that one's last words can be reported back to the home country. This practice is extremely important since the dying person will join 'the world of the ancestors' and will protect the family. Mourning is a means of expressing sadness, and the period of mourning is very important in order not to offend the ancestors. When someone dies, many members of the community will often come to the hospital to see the person who has died and to cry. This may shock care-givers who have been acutely aware of how alone the person had been during their illness. The Zairian community draws very close when someone dies, with groups of women organizing the mourning and the purchase of a garland of flowers, and funds being raised to repatriate the body (from BF 200 000 to BF 300 000 or US $6.500 to US $10.000).

After the death of patients we are frequently faced with how best to provide for orphans, who are often placed in institutions or with temporary foster families. Members of the community who might wish to take care of these children are faced with complicated administrative procedures, and are often in precarious situations themselves, perhaps because of problems over residence permits, housing, and/or financial situation. Some children may be HIV-positive themselves and must be placed in an environment where they can receive regular care. Remaining family members are often separated when a person dies, and the children are not always placed together in the same institution. African communities in Belgium are at present organizing mutual assistance networks in order to work towards some kind of solution for these children.

Conclusion

In this chapter, it has not been possible to discuss all aspects of the problem. In particular, the situation of families with HIV-positive children needs a great deal more attention. This is a very real problem in African communities in Belgium, and there is no doubt that the community as a whole must be made more aware of it if, in collaboration with support associations and grass-roots organizations, we are to make significant progress.

What I have tried to show here is the importance of a cultural approach in providing care and support for members of migrant communities. We have seen how they have specific needs, linked to culture, but also, and above all, how their precarious living conditions and vulnerability will have just as much effect on their ability to gain access to care. An essential and inherent part of the prevention process will be to allow all people living with HIV or AIDS to gain access to care, regardless of colour, religion or culture.

References

BENSALAH, N. (Ed.) (1994) *Familles Turques et Maghrébines Aujourd'hui*, Paris: Maison Neuve-Larose.

BIDEAU, G. (1991) 'L'Afrique terre imaginaire du Sida: La subversion du discours scientifique par le jeu des fantasmes', *Anthropologie et Société*.

CARAËL, M. (1987) 'En Afrique une maladie culturelle', Interview by HIRSCH, E. in *Le Sida: Rumeurs et Faits*, pp. 50–66, Paris: Editions du Cerf.

COURTEJOIE, J. (1987) *Le Sida Est Là, Que Faire?*, Kinshasa: Bureau d'études et de recherche pour la promotion de la santé.

COURTEJOIE, J. and MBOTO, P. (1995) *Le sida et la Famille*, Kinshasa: Bureau d'études et de recherche pour la promotion de la santé.

EHRHASDT, N., DEFOURNY, J. and BERTRAND, J. (1995) *Sida, Pays en Voie de Développement et Ethnopsychiatrie*', Liège: Revue Médicale.

HUBERT, M. (1990) *Sexual Behaviour and Risk of HIV Infection*, Brussels: Université St Louis.

JENARD, H. and CLAEYS-BOUAERT, T. (1988) '*Soins de Santé et Pratiques du Ramadam*', Brussels: Les cahiers du GERM.

JODELET, D. (1988) *Les Représentations Sociales*, Paris: PUF.

PIOT, P. and BILA, K. (1993) '*Sida en Afrique, Manuel du Praticien*', Genève: Organisation Mondiale de la Santé.

PIOT, P. and TEZZO, R. (1990) 'The epidemiology of HIV and other sexually transmitted infections in the developing world', *Scandinavian Journal of Infectious Diseases*, Suppl. 69, pp. 89–97.

SCHOEPF, B.G. (1991) 'Représentation du sida et pratiques populaires à Kinshasa', *Anthropologie et Société*.

Service Social des Etrangers, L'unité du RESO/UCL, Petits Pas (1994) *Etudes et Moyens de Communication Appropriés à la Prévention du Sida dans la Communauté Zaïroise de Belgique*, Brussels: SSE.

TEZZO, R. and PIOT, P. (1989) 'Epidémiologie de l'infection à VIH en zone tropicale', in M. ROSENHEIM, *Sida, Infection à VIH: Aspects en Zone Tropicale*, pp. 48–59, Paris: Editions Ellipses/Aupelf.

Chapter 11

Culture in the Clinic:
Danish Service Providers' View of Immigrants with HIV

Steffen Jöhncke

From his work in a hospital ward caring for people living with HIV, a Danish health professional recalls the following events in his contact with an African woman with HIV living in Denmark. The woman was a widow and had a number of children:

> The children would become orphans at some stage, and we [the hospital staff] wanted to intervene together with the social services at an early stage, and secure a foster-family. A support family to begin with, who then later could take over the children. And then, I do think the social services are very good. They report here with a psychologist and a caseworker, and then we try to talk with the patient about it . . . It has been difficult with those black women, because either they think that they are going to die now, or they think that we take the children away because they [the women] have AIDS. There have been some very long, tough rounds where they have been sitting slap up against the wall with such big, frightened eyes. It has been horrible.

How can it go so wrong? How can the service provider with the best of intentions and access to resources produce such a disastrous effect? In this particular case, the misunderstandings were eventually sorted out, but how can such situations be avoided? Obviously the problem is one of failure of communication between the service provider and the patient. But there is more to it than that. In order to fully understand the background for this event, it is necessary to look at the conditions and problems of service provision to immigrants living with HIV in Denmark.

This chapter is based on a study of service provision to immigrants living with HIV in Denmark. It was carried out by the author in various periods during 1993–5.[1] The aims of the study were, first, to establish an overview of the current situation, based on policy documents and interviews with more than fifty informants, and second to do an in-depth study of particular problems in the field, predominantly based on qualitative interviews with thirty service providers within medical services, support services for people with HIV, and immigrant services. The idea of the latter part of the study was to examine the experiences and views of service providers working with immigrants with HIV, in order to problematize, not the immigrants, but the service providers' approach to immigrant care.

Here the term 'service providers' is taken to mean health professionals — including medical doctors, nurses, social workers, various types of counsellors, as well as administrators — whose work includes the provision of services to immigrants with HIV. The English term 'immigrant' is used here as the nearest equivalent of the Danish word *udlænding*, a person from abroad. Which persons and groups were to be covered by this term was not decided beforehand, as it was part of the study to investigate which criteria service providers used to discern Danish from non-Danish service users. In practice, reference is made both to migrants and members of ethnic minority communities. However, most of the persons concerned are actual immigrants in the sense of having migrated into Denmark in the course of their own lifetime.

The Policy Context

According to Danish law, all persons with legal residence in Denmark have equal and free access to medical and social services. With very few exceptions these services belong to the public sector and are financed through general taxation. Linguistically and culturally, Denmark has a very homogeneous population, and less than 4 per cent of its inhabitants are foreign residents. Nevertheless immigrant communities, especially from Turkey, Pakistan and the former Yugoslavia, together with refugees from many different countries, have been present in the country since the end of the 1960s. On this basis alone one could expect Danish health and social service to have well-developed policies and practices of providing for people whose backgrounds are not Danish. But that is not the case. Rather it is a principle of Danish policy that special provision for, and consideration of, different groups should be minimized. This is usually done with reference to the principle of 'equal treatment', which interestingly is being interpreted in general as 'the same treatment of all', regardless of manifest differences between people.

The principles of equality and unity ('one system for all') can be found both in relation to HIV/AIDS-policy and regarding services to minority ethnic communities. In the 1980s, the AIDS epidemic did give rise to a number of new initiatives in terms of both prevention and care — such as hotlines, special home-support programmes, and a recreational home for people with AIDS. In the 1990s there has been an increasing pressure from both policy makers and the medical establishment to *normalize* HIV/AIDS, and thus to refrain from developing any special provisions in this field. This debate concerning specialization versus the integration or 'normalization' of HIV-related services is not particular to Denmark, as it is found in many countries (Council of Europe, 1992). As a symbolic policy marker, normalization has no fixed content. In some contexts it refers to the end of discrimination and the incorporation of concerns about HIV in everyday life (Campbell, 1995), but in Danish HIV-discourse normalization means adapting people with HIV to the health service, not the other way round. To quote two often-used phrases in this respect, the aim is to 'regard HIV as a disease like any other', to be dealt with 'within the framework of existing services'.

In a parallel fashion, *integration* is the omnipresent buzz word regarding Danish policy towards immigrants. Again, some special provisions have been set up — such as statutory counselling services for ethnic minorities in larger cities, and interpretation services — but the general tendency goes against specialization and towards integration (Henriksen, 1987; Bruun and Hammer, 1993). The question of specialization versus integration is a general issue in health policy towards immigrants in many countries (Bollini, 1993) — Denmark has clearly opted for the latter approach. Characteristically, in Denmark the use of interpreters in medical and social services is not a right for the service user, but an option for the professional service provider. In the interviews of the study on which this chapter is based, there was frequent mention of problems related to the underuse of interpreting services.

The combined effect of 'normalization' and 'integration' is that — beyond the general aim of treating everybody 'equally' — no special objectives, guidelines, or systematic considerations have been adopted anywhere concerning service provision to immigrants living with HIV in Denmark. Both HIV-related services and services to ethnic minority groups are the task of the standard health and social service system, and therefore they are 'everybody's responsibility' in general. Service providers are expected to be able to deal with issues relating both to HIV/AIDS and to ethnic minorities. However, this expectation in itself gives the individual service provider little guidance about how to solve questions and problems that arise in practice. In effect, services to immigrants living with HIV become 'nobody's responsibility' in particular. The individual staff person is left largely to sort out the problems on his or her own, as general inadequacies of policy appear in the everyday practice of social and clinical work. In the interviews there is ample evidence of individual service providers who struggle to provide adequate services, but — as the opening quotation illustrated — they are not always succesful. In this situation, service providers' understanding of the challenge at hand is crucial for the chances of improving conditions and quality of services. Therefore this issue deserves further critical examination.

Service Providers' Understanding of the Problem

Of course not all encounters between Danish professional service providers and immigrants with HIV end up disastrously. There are many accounts of successful contacts, and in the interviews several of the providers explain how they continuously develop their work by learning from past experience. But problems of contact and communication are still mentioned frequently in all interviews. Language problems and lack of interpreting were touched upon above, but beyond the problems of basic verbal understanding, a number of other problems are experienced by the service providers in their work with immigrants living with HIV. These problems are generally presented as *characterizations* of the immigrants — descriptions of particular traits that according to the service staff impede their work and render contact in general difficult. The point here is that these characterizations of immigrants tell a great deal more about the service providers themselves than about the immigrants. Exactly *what* they tell, we shall return to below.

Immigrants living with HIV in Denmark come from all parts of the world, with Africans and Europeans as the largest groups.[2] Therefore, it is not surprising that the service providers often initially point out that 'immigrants' are so diverse as to defy generalization. However, certain characterizations keep appearing in the interviews as regular *markers of difference* between Danes and non-Danes. Especially what makes many immigrants different from most Danes — in the eyes of the service providers — is the immigrants' 'closedness', their sexuality, their way of using services, and their perspectives on disease and death. Under these general headlines, even diametrically opposed examples are mentioned in the interviews with reference to different ethnic groups.

Virtually all of the service providers interviewed agree that generally the immigrants are more 'closed' about their HIV status than Danes who are HIV positive. They report that many immigrants do not tell anyone about their status, and that they do not want to talk with service providers about their situation. On the other hand, some immigrants are reported to be *too* open: 'They tell anyone who cares to listen,' as one service provider said. The Danish staff consider such openness unwise.

Concerning sexuality, the following statement is fairly typical of the interviews, with reference to certain immigrants: 'People from those cultures are not used to talk about sex, in the way that we are.' On the other hand, while many immigrants seem disinclined to talk about sex, some apparently have no problem practising it (still according to the interviews): 'And then their way of life! They are allowed to sleep with anyone, even when they are married.'

Furthermore, according to several interviews many immigrants are not used to having access to services, and they have brought with them from their home country a distrust of authorities. Also, many do not understand how to make claims in the right way: 'They don't say anything, they just sit there [in the clinic]. They don't make any demands.' Or the opposite: some of them make a lot of demands. They have some demands sometimes that make you think: 'This can't be true!'

The final example chosen here concerns perspectives on disease and death. Here too the Danish service providers present a number of characteristics of various immigrants. Many have the impression that some immigrants do not really understand that they are infected with HIV. According to the interviewees, this problem is related to cultural predispositions rather than to insufficient counselling and information: 'Because of his culture the patient can't understand that you can be ill [infected], when you are well.' The idea here is that 'culture' stands in the way of a scientifically correct understanding of the virus. On the other hand, some immigrants demand too much from science, as quoted in one interview: 'They [scientists] have invented pills against everything — why not this as well?' By contrast, as some Danish service providers see it, religious beliefs may be a comfort to some immigrants confronted with death: 'While the Danes intellectualize death, the immigrants from Muslim countries regard death more as a part of life.' On the other hand, religious beliefs can take people too far towards fatalism: 'Allah decides everything. It is very difficult to make a person understand that we don't believe that Allah decides everything, and that certain things we decide ourselves.'

These various characterizations of immigrants illustrate the service providers' understanding of why communication and work with immigrants are so difficult in many instances. But the descriptions of immigrants not only indicate specific problems as the service providers see them — they also point towards the one, fundamental *explanation* of all the problems: immigrants' cultural backgrounds. As one of the interviewees sums it up: 'It's that culture of theirs — that's where the barrier is.'

Whose Culture?

Culture explains everything: this understanding is absolutely dominant in the interviews. Immigrants are considered 'carriers of culture' — not unlike 'carriers of virus': immigrants are culturally different from Danes, and culture sits like an ingrained and unchangeable element within them. In social or clinical work this 'culture of theirs' becomes a 'barrier': the Danish professionals cannot achieve what they consider necessary and good for the patient/client. When difficulties are believed to be the inevitable outcome of immigrants' cultural backgrounds, all problems are systematically placed with the immigrants, and the service providers and the system they represent are exempt from any responsibility.

It is tempting to write off the characterizations of immigrants simply as products of prejudice and racism, and conclude that Danish health and social service professionals need training and better information. Certainly prejudice and racism are present, but to stop at that would not nearly take us far enough towards analysing the problem. In fact, 'better information' might be part of the problem rather than part of the solution, if the question of culture is not addressed properly.

The focus on 'culture' in the interviews is not particular to the service providers. In his analysis of the discourse on immigrants in Danish society, Scandinavian social scientist Carl-Ulrik Schierup (1993) concludes that:

> 'Culture' has . . . become one of the most used and misused free-floating concepts which time and again is taken as an explanation of the problems that ethnic minorities face in society. Many basically social and political questions have been 'explained' in stereotypical cultural terms — they have become *culturalized.* (Schierup, 1993, p. 15)

Likewise, 'culture' has increasingly become central in the understanding of HIV/AIDS as a social phenomenon (Herdt, 1992). On the one hand, cultural approaches have proved useful in the planning and implementation of effective prevention efforts (Bolton and Singer, 1992), when 'culture' is understood as a dynamic and continuous process of cultural change. On the other hand, 'Culture can be used to stigmatize groups as well' (Herdt, 1992, p. 9). This is possible when 'culture' stiffens into a reified image of the alleged lifestyle and behaviour of a particular group. This has been particularly dominant in the epidemiological definition of risk groups for HIV:

> . . . the logic of attributing lethal diseases to those perceived as culturally different became ensconced in the language of 'risk groups'. Individuals defined as members of particular risk groups have come to be seen as at risk because of what are presumed to be their cultural behaviors. (Glick-Schiller *et al.*, 1994, p. 1339)

The idea of risk groups described here also appears in several of the interview quotations above. It appears too that culture is evoked not just in consideration of risk of infection, but also in relation to the provision of care and support for those already infected. Culture stands in the way of services — Frankenberg (1992, p. 7) uses the term 'ethnic non-compliance' to refer to this view: 'These Foreigners are unhealthy because they will not do as we wisely advise; that is because their culture inhibits and prevents them.'

To analyse this culturalized view of risk groups and patients, we need to ask questions about the 'viewers', as it were: How and by whom is this view maintained? Which are the political and — indeed — cultural systems that produce this understanding (Treichler, 1992)? The culturalization of immigrants with HIV is attractive to the service providers in this study because it neutralizes and obscures the political character of the blame and criticism directed at the service users. 'Culture is not a politically neutral concept,' as Glick-Schiller *et al.* (1994, p. 1344) remind us — culture is part of the politics of AIDS, as reified images of culture are used as one of the means to discern between 'them' and 'us'. Since 'The politics of AIDS, as gay men, people of color, and others have experienced directly, is a politics of division, stigmatization, and moral blame' (Singer, 1994, p. 1321), therefore: 'AIDS presents ... a sort of social X-ray of who is classified as mainstream and peripheral, deviant and normal' (Herdt, 1992, pp. 8–9).

Some of the interesting questions raised by service providers' descriptions and judgments of the immigrants include the following: since service providers have the power of definition, what are the norms, values and ideals that the immigrants are compared to? What are the cultural prescriptions that patients and clients are expected to live up to? Or put in another way: what is expected of a patient in the culture of the clinic? Analysing the interviews in this light, the material often gives a very detailed account of the *ideal* patient/client. Taking here only the statements presented above, the following outline appears: the ideal patient is 'open' and shows confidence and trust in the service provider, but is careful about openness to others. The ideal patient understands and appreciates conversation as an integral part of services to people with HIV. The ideal patient is open to talking about sexual matters with the service provider, but is modest in sexual practices. The ideal patient shows trust in authorities and demands exactly what the service system can deliver (no more, no less). The ideal patient understands and accepts only scientific definitions of HIV/AIDS, and at the same times demands no more than that which medical science can deliver. The ideal patient might be religious, but only so far as this does not interfere with being 'responsible' for himself and 'rational' about death.

Of course, many Danish service users are likely to come into conflict with this ideal role too. But because of language problems and a higher degree of unfamiliarity with the Danish health and social service system, immigrants are more likely to deviate from the norms defined by the Danish service providers. Immigrant patients are less likely to negotiate an impression and present a behaviour that will satisfy the role ascribed to a user of the Danish social and health services.

Out of the Culture Trap

The service providers are not simply anti-immigrant — actually most of them are deeply worried about the situation and are keen to improve services to immigrants. To begin with, the problem is that they look the wrong way for solutions: they don't think they know enough about the immigrants' cultural backgrounds to be able to understand and be of more help. If immigrants' culture is believed to explain all difficulties, the solution to the problem follows naturally: virtually all of the service providers want more knowledge about immigrants' cultures. Often they request detailed information about traditions, beliefs and norms in the various cultures from which immigrants come. This, they believe, will explain why the immigrants do as they do. The service providers want to live up to what they think is expected of them as professionals: they want to understand their patients and clients.

However attractive it is to gain knowledge of different cultures, few of the service providers realize what an enormous project this is. With the sheer number of different ethnic groups represented in Denmark, and the endless row of potentially relevant cultural facts to be mapped out — regarding family life, kinship, gender, sexuality, religion, food, disease, death, etc. — there is enough to keep anyone permanently occupied. One service provider gave the following account of how she and a group of colleagues attempted to develop their own catalogue of cultures:

> Each of us took a language or a culture, and made an interview with a person from that area. After I don't know how many interviews, we agreed that it wasn't possible. It is not that simple . . . Many things were the same, [but] in the end we couldn't find any similarities, without having to do even more work. An enormous task! So we dropped it after having worked with it for quite a long time.
>
> But — no, it depends on a humility on the part of the [professional] person, . . . [who] must try to find out . . . well, what is the situation of the person [the service user] now? And all the time try to have a bit of sensitivity about the person in front of you.

This group of staff learned from their own experience that 'knowledge of immigrants' cultures' is not exactly gained in a rush. Moreover, the question remains how applicable this knowledge will be in practice. This is not to deny that general insights into other cultures might provide useful guidelines, but it never renders superfluous learning directly from the individual in question himself or herself. Only he or she knows his or her own story and present conditions. Cultures are shared systems of values, norms and ideas — but a person is never just an automatic pawn living out the dictates of a culture: no one is only a 'culture carrier'. Focusing too much on 'knowledge of cultures' runs the risk of cultural reification and stereotyping, which in itself creates barriers for service provision as the individual perspective is lost. But even worse, insisting that only more knowledge of immigrants' culture can solve the present problems is also a good way of doing nothing at all. If changes are postponed until enough knowledge has been collected, the changes will never happen: there is after all always more to learn. The best source of more knowledge is the one at hand: to ask the person himself or herself.

The attempt to explain problems in contact and communication only with immigrants' cultural backgrounds suffers from a double inadequacy: the focus is on only one of the parties (the immigrant), and only on his or her past (background). *A better solution must involve both parties and consider the situation here and now.* Cultural systems give shape and meaning to the life and experiences of individuals. The dominant culture of a person's environment shape his or her basic values and beliefs, but that does not mean that they never change. Migrants are the obvious example of persons whose life courses and experiences have demanded adaptation and change. Therefore it is entirely misleading to ask about migrants' cultural *backgrounds*, and ignore the conditions under which they are presently living.

A few of the service providers interviewed do express an alternative understanding of the problems at hand. First they focus on the total social situation of the individual immigrant, including crucial questions such as his or her current social network (or lack thereof), economic conditions and psychological state. They try to understand the situation of being an immigrant in Denmark, not least in terms of how to work with unfamiliar bureaucracies of health and social services. Some service providers are very critical of these bureaucracies and the way immigrants are treated here. They do not explain distrust in authorities with the immigrants' *past* but to their *present*: how do Danish authorities treat immigrants? Some are also critical of the insufficient resources and time allocated to provide care and support for immigrants, including the underuse of interpreters and bicultural staff. The bottom line in these considerations is that conditions in the health and social service systems are brought out as part of the problem. Whereas a focus on 'cultural background' systematically places the roots of all problems with the immigrants, the broader view of the problems traces inadequacies in Danish policies and bureaucracies, the working conditions of service providers, as well as the immigrant's social and economic situation in Denmark here and now. All of these factors shape the problems to be solved, and consequently all must be addressed in the attempt to provide adequate services to immigrants living with HIV. At the very least, the professionals must begin to direct their criticism towards the policies and systems of service provision that they themselves represent, rather than continue to blame the immigrants who are subjected to these very policies and systems.

In some countries, there is a large enough population basis for having separate services targeting specific minority ethnic communities (O'Brien, 1993). Elsewhere, like in Denmark, where immigrants are few and at the same time ethnically very diverse, particular HIV/AIDS service agencies for each community are unrealistic. What is both possible and essential, though, is that minority ethnic organizations be supported to work with HIV, and AIDS service organizations likewise to work with immigrants and ethnic communities. Still, the general public social and health sector is likely to continue to be the main provider of services to immigrants living with HIV in Denmark. Therefore, staff from these services need to broaden their understanding of the many factors and problems potentially involved in living with HIV in a foreign country, and they need to develop a more useful concept of culture.

Culture begins at home. The best starting point for understanding other people's cultures is to appreciate that you have a culture yourself. Service providers need to look critically at their own norms and values, and how they influence their perception of patients and clients. Immigrants offer an exceptionally good opportunity for bringing these norms and values out in the open. If service providers want to, they have a chance to reflect critically on their relationship to all service users. They also have a chance to develop a *general* cultural sensitivity and thus be better equipped to discuss with the individual patient/client how to appreciate and accommodate cultural differences in the process of service provision.

Notes

1 The study was financed by the European Commission (General Directorate V), Sygekassernes Helsefond (Denmark), and HIV-Danmark (the national organization of people living with HIV), where the project was also based. The results of study are published more fully in Jöhncke (1995). The author is responsible for the study and its conclusions, and the funders do not necessarily share the opinions expressed here.
2 Available epidemiological evidence (from Statens Seruminstitut, Copenhagen) shows that in the period August 1990 to December 1994, 22.6 per cent of all persons testing positive for HIV in Denmark were counted as 'immigrant or refugee' (331 out of 1 462); 65 per cent of the immigrants with HIV came from Sub-Saharan Africa, with Europeans as the second largest group (18.4 per cent).

References

BOLLINI, P. (1993) 'Health for immigrants and refugees in the 1990s: A comparative study in seven receiving countries', *Innovation in Social Sciences Research*, **6**, 1, pp. 101–10.

BOLTON, R. and SINGER, M. (Eds) (1992) *Rethinking AIDS Prevention: Cultural Approaches*, Philadelphia: Gordon & Breach Science Publishers.

BRUUN, I. and HAMMER, O. (1993) 'Brændpunkter i dansk indvandrer- og flygtningepolitik 1993' (Focal points in Danish Policy on Immigrants and Refugees 1993), *Dokumentation om Indvandrere,* **4**, Copenhagen: Mellemfolkeligt Samvirke.

CAMPBELL, I. (1995) 'Moving from fear to hope', in REID, E. (Ed.) *HIV and AIDS: The Global Inter-connection,* West Hartford: Kumarian Press.

COUNCIL OF EUROPE (1992) *Impact of the Aids Epidemic on Health Care Services in Europe,* Strasbourg: Council of Europe Publishing and Documentation Service.

FRANKENBERG, R. (1992) 'What identity's at risk?: Anthropologists and AIDS', in *Anthropology in Action,* **12**.

GLICK-SCHILLER, N., CRYSTAL, S. and LEWELLEN, D. (1994) 'Risky business: The cultural construction of AIDS risk groups', *Social Science and Medicine,* **38**, 10, pp. 1337–46.

HENRIKSEN, I. (1987) *Mødet Mellem Indvandrerfamilier og Social- og Sundhedsvæsenet* (The encounter between immigrant families and the social and health services), **158**, Copenhagen: Socialforskningsinstituttet.

HERDT, G. (1992) 'Introduction', in HERDT, G. and LINDENBAUM, S. (Eds) *The Time of AIDS: Social Analysis, Theory, and Method,* Newbury Park: Sage.

JÖHNCKE, S. (1995) *Hvis Kultur?: Politik og Praksis i Indsatsen for HIV-smittede Udlændinge i Danmark* (Whose Culture?: Politics and practices in service provision to immigrants living with HIV in Denmark), Copenhagen: HIV-Danmark.

O'BRIEN, O. (1993) *Assessing the Impact of HIV on the Irish Community in Britain: An Examination of Current Issues and Service Provision,* London: Positively Irish Action on AIDS.

SCHIERUP, C-U. (1993) *På Kulturens Slagmark: Mindretal og Størretal Taler om Danmark* (In the Battlefield of Culture: Minorities and Majorities Speak of Denmark), Esbjerg: Sydjysk Universitetsforlag.

SINGER, M. (1994) 'Introduction: The politics of AIDS', *Social Science and Medicine,* **38**, 10, pp. 1321–4.

TREICHLER, P.A. (1992) 'AIDS, HIV and the cultural construction of reality', in HERDT, G. and LINDENBAUM, S. (Eds) *The Time of AIDS: Social Analysis, Theory, and Method,* Newbury Park: Sage.

Chapter 12

Asylum Seekers and Clandestine Populations

Alberto Matteelli and Issa El-Hamad

An increase in migratory flow has generated political debate and moral concern at a time when countries in western Europe, which had been receptive to migration, are experiencing economic recession and rising unemployment. The energy crisis of the 1970s can be identified as the historical moment at which a change took place in attitude towards labour immigration in many countries, a change followed by common and coordinated interventions for members of the European community to restrict immigration flows. With the Schengen agreement of 1990, Germany, France, Belgium, The Netherlands, Italy, Spain, Greece, Portugal and Luxembourg chose to effect more severe immigration control at airports and borders, as a prerequisite for the free circulation of residents within their boundaries. The agreement, translated into national laws on 22 December 1994 in most of these countries (except Italy and Greece), points to a common and restrictive political response to problems of migration. Along the same lines, the Dublin convention of 3 June 1991 established an extension of the rights of host countries in the European Community to deny refugee status to asylum seekers. Furthermore, on 20 June 1994 the Ministers of Internal Affairs of the EU countries approved more restrictive rules for employment of non-EU citizens who, in practical terms, could obtain a job only on the basis of a temporary contract. The political picture summarized above, and specifically the decision to limit the forms that legal immigration can take, has led to an increase in clandestine immigration into the community area.

Magnitude of Illegal Migration

There are two categories of legally unrecognized immigrants in European countries. 'Irregular residents' are those who enter the country with a regular permit and eventually remain beyond the limits of the permission granted. Asylum seekers belong to this category when, following refusal of asylum, they decide to remain irregularly in the country. 'Clandestine' migrants, the second category, decide to enter and stay in the country without a regular visa. A special case is that of asylum seekers awaiting decision on or appealing their requests. In most European countries their social rights are granted for an initial period of a few months, after which their position becomes unclear and ambiguous.

The number of individuals seeking asylum in European countries has risen sharply since the mid-1980s: fourteen western European countries report a linear increase from 12 000 in 1972 to 75 000 in 1983, and more than 200 000 annually since 1986 (Hendriks, 1991). This main reason for the increase in asylum applications is likely to be, as mentioned above, the tightening of restrictions to labour immigration: individuals who would previously have entered a country as labour migrants now enter as asylum seekers. As the number of refusals to grant refugee status is also increasing,[1] it is conceivable that many of those asylum seekers refused remain in the country as clandestine migrants. In Switzerland for example, 37 000 requests for asylum were examined in 1991, of which 28 000 (77 per cent) were rejected (Office Fédéral des Réfugiés, 1992). Half of the asylum seekers could not later be traced, a large proportion of whom may be considered to have become clandestine.

Thus the number of clandestine migrants is also increasing, despite the efforts of EU countries to coordinate and tighten their immigration policies, and possibly because of them. Precise calculations as to the exact numbers are not possible for obvious reasons, but estimates of clandestine residents in some European countries, compared with the total number of regular immigrant residents, are reported in Table 12.1 (Geraci, 1995). The proportion of clandestine in relation to regular immigrants is higher in southern European countries such as Spain and Italy than in northern countries. This is likely to be related to the fact that in southern countries immigration is a recent, rapidly expanding phenomenon, and that these areas have recently attracted waves of labour migration. Southern countries, in addition, have relatively limited experience and legal background on immigration policies and are therefore more accessible to clandestine immigration.

Socio-demographic Characteristics and Basic Health Problems

Some of the characteristics differentiating clandestine migrants from those with regular status are summarized in Table 12.2. The socio-economic

Table 12.1 Number of regular immigrants and estimated number of clandestine migrants in selected European countries, 1993

Country	Population (2)	Regular Immigrants (1)	Clandestine Migrants (1)	Ratio Clandestine/Regulars
Belgium	10 068 000	920 000	600 000	0.65
Denmark	5 180 000	170 000	60 000	0.35
France	56 652 000	3 500 000	2 000 000	0.57
Germany	80 975 000	6 000 000	2 000 000	0.33
Italy	56 960 000	980 000	800 000	0.81
Luxembourg	400 000	128 000	120 000	0.93
Spain	39 048 000	360 000	500 000	1.39
The Netherlands	15 239 000	734 000	600 000	0.82
United Kingdom	57 222 000	2 000 000	230 000	0.12

Source: 1 Geraci, 1995
2 Eurostat, 1994

Table 12.2   Characteristics of regular migrants and clandestine migrants

	Regular Migrants	Clandestine Migrants
Socio-economic conditions	depending on level of integration	poor
Environmental health risks	variable	high
Legal rights to health system	present	absent
Access to health system	difficult	very difficult
Type of health services	public health system	voluntary organizations
Coverage of health services	high	low and scattered

conditions of clandestine migrants are often at the lowest limit of the range for migrants in general, while environmental health risks are the highest. Clandestine migrants have no legally recognized rights to health security, and their access to health services is extremely limited, confined to organizations available in the voluntary sector.

Epidemiological data on clandestine migrants are scanty, heterogeneous and jeopardized by the fact that only local observational studies are available, while epidemiological characteristics may vary widely both between countries and within regions in a country. Even when useful information is gained in the course of a study, dissemination is often a problem. Data collected since 1983 by Caritas in Rome has provided information on more than 30 000 attendants to health clinics for immigrants (Geraci, 1995). Although data have not been stratified by legal status, a significant proportion of the attendants are thought to be clandestine migrants. That immigration is an extremely dynamic phenomenon in this setting is demonstrated by the variability in the origin of the immigrants: at the beginning of the 1980s, Africans predominated, coming from Egypt, Somalia, Ethiopia and Senegal. They were replaced by eastern Europeans in the late 1980s (47 per cent of the total in 1986, mainly from Poland and Yugoslavia), then by Africans again (from the horn of Africa) and immigrants from Asia (Bangladesh and Pakistan) in 1990, by eastern Europeans (Albania and Romania) one year later, and, most recently, by Latin Americans. As for gender, males were largely predominant in the first years, though female attendance increased up to a maximum of 48 per cent in 1993. Male–female ratios differ significantly by ethnic group: males predominate among north Africans and south-east Asians, while 71 per cent and 61 per cent of Latin Americans and Somali clinic attenders are females. There has recently been an increase in the number of children among attenders, many of whom are born in the host country, an indication of willingness to integrate into the new society. Roughly half of the subjects report having obtained secondary education, but up to 60 per cent are unemployed or hold unskilled jobs and earn very low salaries. About 60 per cent of the individuals were reported to share their accommodation with one or, more frequently, many friends.

Similar to what is observed in migrants in general, clandestine migrants are in basically good health on arrival. However, a number of problems eventually arise, most of which are poverty related and acquired in the host country. According to Caritas case records in Rome (Geraci, 1995), most attenders in 1993 presented with gastro-intestinal (11.6 per cent), respiratory tract (11.3 per cent), and orthopaedic problems (10.3 per cent). Obstetric and gynaecological consultations were also frequent (9 per cent). Although concern for immigrants' health is most often directed towards communicable parasitic diseases of exotic origin, a specific infectious disease was diagnosed in only 7.8 per cent of the attenders: tuberculosis was most frequently identified, along with sexually transmitted diseases such as syphilis and gonorrhoea. Finally, a consistent proportion of consultations were grouped in the category of psychological disorders, linked to the migratory event, lack of a job, lack of a stable income, or the unavailability of family support.

Clandestine Populations and Risk of HIV/STD

There are no data to suggest that the incidence of HIV infection and AIDS among immigrants is higher than that among local populations. Similarly, whether clandestine migrants present higher risks of HIV/AIDS than migrants in general has never been investigated in controlled studies. Determining rates of HIV or AIDS in migrants in general, and among clandestine migrants in particular, is characterized by the difficulties in determining denominators and, therefore, by a high probability of error. A possible source of data is the national notification system for AIDS cases. In Italy the proportion of immigrants among notified AIDS cases showed a modest increase from 2.2 per cent in 1986 to 4.3 per cent in 1994 (COA, 1995). This figure must be compared with the 2–5 per cent proportion of immigrants in the total resident population (which also presents an increasing trend). Cases among immigrants differ from others in that they showed a higher proportion of bisexual (38 per cent vs 13 per cent) and heterosexual (32 per cent vs 8 per cent) contact as the probable route of infection. In Belgium, HIV transmission patterns also differ between immigrant and local populations: heterosexual transmission accounts for 70 per cent of the AIDS cases in the migrant community of Sub-Saharan origin, while male homosexual transmission is responsible for 80 per cent of the cases in Belgians (Dienst Epidemiologie, 1990). In Denmark roughly 8 per cent of notified AIDS cases are among migrants, while less than 4 per cent of people living in Denmark are so. However, migrants accounted for just over 20 per cent of people testing HIV positive in the period 1990–94 (Rector, 1994). Although the reasons for this contrast are unclear, it may be realistic to expect the proportion of foreigners among people with AIDS to increase within the next few years. Alternative sources of epidemiological information are sometimes available, such as the national STD surveillance system in Italy. Though legal and illegal immigrants are not differentiated, clandestine migrants are likely to be over-represented among clinic attenders, as services are delivered anonymously. In almost 2 000 immigrants tested from 1990 to 1994, HIV prevalence was 5.7 per cent (Giuliani and Suligoi, 1995). In comparison, HIV prevalence rates in the overall attending populations was 9.3 per cent (Suligoi *et al.*, 1994), thus higher than that of migrants. The probability of a positive HIV test was poorly related to HIV prevalence in the general population of the home country, and highly associated with individual behaviour, mainly sexual activity (Gattari *et al.*, 1992).

As shown in the figures presented above, migrants are likely to be particularly vulnerable to the risk of sexual transmission of HIV. Migrant sex workers deserve special attention in this regard. The number of migrants offering sexual services in Europe is increasing considerably, a phenomenon due both to migration itself and to the exploitation of sexual traffic organized to meet the demand for low-priced prostitution. In European cities where registered prostitution is legal, unregistered prostitutes, most of whom are migrants, often outnumber the registered ones (Mardh and Genc, 1995). Though many of them (i.e. those from eastern Europe) may come from areas where the prevalence of HIV is lower than in western Europe, they may be at increased risk of STDs and HIV for several reasons. First, many are non-professional: this may increase the risks of STDs due to reduced awareness of potential health risks and of effective protective measures. A recent study of Romanian sex workers in Istanbul, for example, revealed that 28 per cent of the girls were first-time prostitutes, with very low awareness of STDs (Genc *et al.*, 1993). Second, migrant sex workers, both males and females, sell sexual services in order to survive or to gain financial stability, and may be prepared to incur very high risks for their health because of their difficult economic situation. Finally, clandestine sex workers very seldom come in contact with health-care providers and therefore derive minimal benefits from public preventive and curative health services. Parental transmission of HIV due to injecting drug use may also be an important risk in some immigrant populations. South American transsexual sex workers in Rome present high prevalence rates of HIV which were significantly associated with injecting drug use (Spizzichino, 1993).

There are no data to answer the question whether HIV-positive individuals migrate with the HIV infection or acquire it in the host country, though this information would be of value in order to organize targeted interventions for prevention. Spizzichino's (1993) study of transsexual sex workers showed an increase in both sex- and drug-related risk behaviour since residency in Italy, indicating the possibility that HIV may be acquired, at least in part, in the host country.

Medical Screening among Asylum Seekers and HIV Testing

By definition, no medical screening or testing can be performed of clandestine migrants on their entry into the host country. Organized medical screening programmes do, on the contrary, exist for some asylum seekers entering a receiving country, examples of which are provided in Sweden and Switzerland (Bollini, 1992). Although screening on entry can by no means be a substitute for continual health assistance to the immigrant, a medical consultation at the time of initial entry may be seen as a unique chance to intervene on the health of an individual who may eventually become clandestine and loose all legal rights to health care.

In Switzerland, a decentralized mandatory programme for the screening of asylum seekers was implemented at the cantonal level from 1984 to 1992, and eventually reorganized to have eight registration/transit centres act as central screening sites (Loutan, 1992). The programme is targeted to the early diagnosis of tuberculosis and hepatitis B, to vaccinations according to age group (influenza, measles, mumps, rubella), and to the provision of health information/education, including written information on AIDS transmission. Many drawbacks in the screening system were identified. First, screening is costly and requires a great deal of logistic and managerial capacity. Appropriate pre- and post-counselling facilities are necessary: in the case of hepatitis B infection, for example, this should concern the risk of transmission, the evolution of the disease, and desired changes in behaviour. Finally, immigrants may perceive screening with an attitude of suspicion, and may fear that the detection of any disease will be used to deny asylum, which in turn determines reduced acceptance and poor compliance.

On the other hand, the possible positive role of screening is shown by the potential for prevention of tuberculosis. Tuberculosis is re-emerging as a worldwide problem, and immigrants from highly endemic areas are recognized as a high-risk population in western countries, with a 5–25-fold increase in incidence compared to the local population (Carosi *et al.*, 1993). Tuberculosis among immigrants can be due to both reactivation of latent infection and the acquisition of new pathogens in the community; the migratory event itself is likely to be the triggering factor in both cases, as research shows incidence to peak in the first years after migration. Screening of immigrants, early diagnosis, and chemotherapy have been proposed as cost-effective tools for tuberculosis control in western countries (Spinaci and Aronson, 1990). However, the low acceptance of these measures among migrants has been demonstrated, due to communication barriers, the mobility of the target population and the unavailability of appropriate health infrastructures.

From the available evidence, it is clear that there is no role for HIV testing among screening procedures for entry, as available epidemiological data on HIV transmission and natural history show that allowing HIV infected migrants into a country does not create additional risk to the local population. Moreover, compulsory testing violates internationally accepted human rights accords. From a financial point of view HIV screening would hardly be sustainable: the identification of groups to be screened would bring unacceptable discrimination among migrants, while screening all arrivals would divert an enormous amount of resources from more cost-effective prevention interventions.

HIV-Related Preventive and Curative Health Care for Clandestine Populations

There is some evidence that migrant populations in general have less knowledge and are probably less aware of the risks involved in certain sexual behaviours (van Duifhuizen, 1990). However, a small questionnaire survey among 200 clandestine migrants in Rome revealed adequate knowledge about HIV/AIDS and its prevention among 62 per cent of the sample, a proportion similar to that frequently observed in students in European countries (Zurlo and Geraci, 1991); education programmes should therefore take into account the fact that safe behaviour may be known about, but difficult to act upon. Effective HIV/AIDS prevention interventions require an understanding of the specific perceptions and needs of the target population. Very little work has so far been done among asylum seekers and clandestine migrants. Despite all constraints, some health education materials for asylum seekers have been developed, for example, videos produced by the Centre for Refugees Health Care in The Netherlands, which are available in sixteen languages (Hendriks, 1991). The International Organisation for Migration (IOM) and United Nations High Commission for Refugees (UNHCR) have also drafted guidelines for the management of AIDS/HIV. There are no examples of similar interventions among clandestine communities.

Very little is known about how best to evaluate interventions among clandestine migrants, but specific challenges arise here as well. Questionnaire surveys and interviews have limited acceptance among clandestine migrants and a high refusal rate may cause biases in the sampling of population groups. Due to their illegal status, clandestine migrants may be induced to give false answers on topics thought to be harmful for their stay in the country. Finally, the high mobility of these groups significantly decreases the feasibility of performing the longitudinal studies which would otherwise be most indicated to evaluate interventions.

The position of clandestine migrants is even weaker in relation to curative health-care services. Since the beginning of the HIV epidemic, assumptions and links have been made between migrants and AIDS, yet very little has been done to improve the quality of services provided for migrants living with or at risk of HIV/AIDS (Rector, 1994). Clandestine migrants seeking medical care may only be able to visit private physicians or clinics run by benevolent organizations. Physician visits, however, are largely limited by economic factors.

Non-governmental organizations (NGOs), religious orders and small voluntary groups have an increasingly significant role in developing community-based information and treatment programmes for clandestine migrants. NGOs have both advantages and disadvantages in comparison with official services. Quantitatively, several shortcomings may be identified: coverage of the clandestine population may be insufficient; coordination and standardization of procedures among different organizations is often unsatisfactory; funds are very often limited, and the duration of established programmes may be uncertain; the range of facilities and specialist services available at voluntary clinics may be much smaller than that of official clinics. Qualitatively, voluntary services may have significant advantages compared to official ones: personnel are often highly motivated and have basic knowledge of the cultural background of the clients resulting in higher acceptance and overall efficacy of services rendered. As a consequence, voluntary clinics for clandestine migrants may also be ideal for outreach interventions in the community at a preventive level.

It is usually felt to be highly unlikely that official services will open their doors to clandestine migrants. In fact, preventive and curative interventions for them would be contradictory from several points of view: helping clandestine migrants may imply complicity between official and illegal bodies, and mismanaged interventions might lead to the individual's expulsion from the country. A further consideration worth mentioning is exemplified by the recent approval in the USA of California's Proposition 187, stating that publicly funded health facilities and physicians should deny non-emergency medical treatment to undocumented or illegal aliens. Some have pointed out that although providing care without compensation is a commendable act, we need to be fully aware that in many instances we are 'playing poker with other people chips', as the salaries and costs of diagnostic procedures and treatment come from institutional or public coffers (Iseman and Starke, 1995). One possibility is for the public health system to play a role in caring for clandestine populations by financing and coordinating the activities of a network of voluntary organizations, thus filling the quantitative gaps of qualitatively adequate structures.

Public Health Services for Clandestine Migrants: The Experience in Brescia

In contrast with the usual circumstances reported above, in some instances the public health system has taken direct responsibility for health-care services

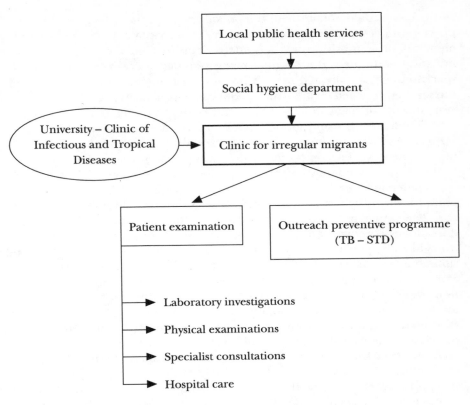

Table 12.3 Clinic for irregular migrants in Brescia: Structure and activities

for clandestine populations. This is the case of Brescia, a small industrial town in the north of Italy. The area has a relatively high proportion of immigrants. Ten thousand are regularly settled and an additional 10 000 are either clandestine migrants or temporarily illegal. Altogether, immigrants represent roughly 2 per cent of the resident population. The local authorities responsible for preventive and curative public health services signed a contract in 1990 which established a clinic (see Table 12.3 for structure and activities) to provide services for immigrants who were waiting to regularize their status. Without it being explicitly stated, the purpose was to extend such services to all clandestine immigrants. Funds were made available to hire consultant physicians, and nursing staff was provided from the public health system. Expertise in the field of migration and health was obtained from the local academic institution rather than from voluntary organizations. The unit was empowered to request most laboratory investigations, basic examinations and specialist consultations. On the basis of an agreement between public health and hospital services, admission to hospital for severe medical conditions was authorized. At the beginning drugs were prescribed and patients could obtain them free, thanks to a special agreement with the pharmacist network. Eighteen months after the service was opened, the agreement for drug provision was terminated due to high costs, but all other initiatives continued, the contract being renewed every year. Although no special budget was created for this initiative, it is estimated that the costs of the services provided by the clinic amount to approximately US $300 000 per year, mostly for haematological tests and routine investigations.

The unit is physically located in a room nextdoor to other public health services. The opening time is every afternoon five days a week; no appointment is needed. The unit aims at delivering basic preventive and curative health services to migrants without other forms of assistance, collecting baseline epidemiological information on health needs, and creating an entry point for the diffusion of educational messages within clandestine communities. The centre also provides information about the administrative procedures for the regularization of immigration status in all cases where this is thought to be possible. From January 1990 to June 1995 almost 15 000 consultations were recorded, of which more than 5 000 were first consultations, with a yearly average of more than 3 000 and 1 000 total and first consultations respectively. The number of consultations dropped in the third trimester of 1992 following the termination of free drug prescription; thereafter a mild increasing trend was observed again. It is estimated that more than 90 per cent of the consultants are clandestine or irregular immigrants. The vast majority arrive from western and northern African countries (mainly Senegal and Morocco). Observations indicate that attenders belong to a recent and still unsettled community: the male–female ratio is 9–1, more than 80 per cent are 20–40 years old, up to 90 per cent live as singles in the host country, and more than 70 per cent have settled for less than two years. The majority (40 per cent) are unemployed, or without a stable job (37 per cent).

The reasons for consultations are similar to those observed for migrants in general, with a large predominance of pathologies acquired in the host country and associated to conditions of poverty and marginalization. Among communicable diseases, tuberculosis is the leading problem, followed by sexually transmitted diseases (STDs). A pilot project for the control of tuberculosis among clandestine migrants was started in 1991, and recently reviewed and modified in order to tackle the major identifiable constraints: low awareness of the importance of medical screening to prevent disease, low compliance to prophylaxis and treatment schedules, high mobility and the scarcity of community leaders. Very recently, another pilot project was designed to tackle the problem of STDs among female clandestine sex workers: it focuses on the collection of epidemiological data, KAPB data, and the pre-testing of information material. HIV screening is not included among routine activities of the clinic for a number of reasons. First, adequate care cannot be granted to those whose test result is positive; second, adequate and appropriate pre-test and post-test counselling to culturally different subjects cannot be offered since skilled and dedicated personnel are not available; and third, there is widespread fear that, despite assurances of confidentiality, data may be used against individuals who are already extremely vulnerable legally.

HIV testing, however, is performed whenever specifically requested by the patient. Testing is also actively advised in some circumstances in which it is considered that being aware of the possible infection would be beneficial for the health of the individual or for public health reasons. This is the case for the following conditions: pregnancy, symptoms suggestive of AIDS, drug abuse and involvement in sex work.

The complexity of the problems arising from the combined occurrence of HIV infection and illegal status is clearly demonstrated by the experience of the few clandestine individuals found to be HIV positive or to have AIDS. Those who are asymptomatic and have no immunological impairment are informed about the infection, its possible progression to disease, and the importance of regular follow-up. A common observation of the service providers is the difficulty of making people understand the severity of the problem and its real consequences for the individual's well-being. Information is also given on routes of transmission and recommended safe behaviours. Here, again, it is felt that the likelihood that individuals will follow recommendations is directly linked to their comprehension of the severity of the problem. Follow-up visits and all necessary examinations are thereafter performed at the clinic itself or, following special agreements, at the local academic institution. No practical solutions are available when chronic treatment becomes necessary: anti-retroviral therapy cannot be obtained from the pharmacies because a prescription reporting details on the public medical code is required. Preventive treatment for common opportunistic infections can be prescribed, but the economic burden of life-long therapy can hardly be sustained by most of the clients. If medicine is somehow provided, compliance to recommended schedules is often poor (due partly to the fact that much preventive treatment is targeted at asymptomatic people). Apart from the medical needs, social and welfare needs are poorly satisfied as well. Individuals who gradually lose their working capabilities have little if any possibility of survival; they usually have no family, and no support can be expected from the social system of the host country. They can only rely on support from their own community, whenever this is not precluded by prejudice about AIDS.

With disease progression, HIV infected individuals need continual assistance as they become unable to care for themselves. They may be admitted to hospital for an acute event, but when discharged they are unable to use public long-term residency facilities where nursing services are available. Taking into consideration the whole range of foreseeable events and the increasing problems a clandestine HIV positive individual will need to face, most service providers advise, if requested, that they return home at the earliest chance. This advice is given in full awareness that 'curative' and diagnostic facilities in the home country may be scarce or non-existent. This, however, is exactly equivalent to what is available to an illegal resident in the host country. In the home country, at least, the chances of obtaining family and social support in a culturally more familiar environment may be higher.

Conclusion

Clandestine immigration into European countries is an expanding phenomenon. Though precise figures are not available, clandestine migrants represent significant proportions of all immigrants, especially in southern European countries. Clandestine migrants cannot be considered a source of HIV infection into the host country. Nor do they represent a group at special risk for HIV *per se*. However, for socio-cultural and economic reasons, subgroups of clandestine migrants may have behaviour patterns that create increased susceptibility to HIV infection. Clandestine immigrants working as sex workers may be exposed to a particularly high risk. Because clandestine migrants live at the margins of society, they are likely to remain unreached by information and education on HIV/AIDS.

Little attention has been given so far to the problems of migrants living with HIV or AIDS, and clandestine migrants are no exception. They have no access to preventive and curative health services from official public health structures. Voluntary organizations often replace official bodies, but they have limited coverage, coordination and financial capacities. People in the initial phases of infection require psychological support from the family, the society, and by social and medical bodies, none of which is usually available. Service providers are still unprepared to provide appropriate social and medical psychological support. People with medium-term HIV infection require medical attention which includes repeated physical examinations, hematological and immunological monitoring, and anti-retroviral therapy, none of which, again, can usually be provided. Those with advanced disease may have pathological conditions which need hospital care. Emergency care is provided in all host countries, but this is unlikely to be consistently guaranteed to individuals affected by chronic disease. Hospitals, moreover, in a climate of increasing severe immigration regulation, may be used as a point for the identification of clandestine migrants.

Whatever our individual political beliefs, we cannot forget that clandestine migrants, as well as a country's other residents, are affected by the HIV/AIDS epidemic. At a minimum, tools to face the problem must include: maintaining the availability of services for urgent medical conditions; providing public and individual health care for infants and pregnant women (on humanitarian grounds); and providing public and individual health care for diseases such as tuberculosis and sexually transmitted diseases/HIV (on public health grounds). It has been said that human pathogens fail to recognize country boundaries. Pathogens also fail to respect inhabitants' legal status.

Note

1 People seeking asylum in European countries may stay permanently only if they are granted refugee status. See the definitions in the introductory chapter to this book.

References

BOLLINI, P. (1992) 'Health policies for immigrant population in the 1990s: A comparative study in seven receiving countries', *International Migration Quarterly Review*, **30**, pp. 103–19.

CAROSI, G., CARVALHO, A.C., MATTEELLI, A., SIGNORINI, L., EL-HAMAD, I. and CASTELLI F. (1993) 'Risk of tuberculosis in international travel and migration', Third Conference on International Travel Medicine, Paris 25–29 April, Abs. 9.

CENTRO OPERATIVO AIDS (1995) 'Aggiornamento dei casi di AIDS notificati in Italia al 31 Dicembre 1994', *Notiziario dell'Instituto Superiore di Sanità*, **8**, 3, pp. 1–15.

DIENST EPIDEMIOLOGIE (1990) 'AIDS epidemiologie en besmetting mit HIV en Belgie: Toestand op 31 December 1989', Brussels: Instituut voor Hygiene en Epidemiologie, November.

VAN DUIFHUIZEN R. (1990) 'AIDS prevention towards migrants in The Netherlands', Country report, National Committee on AIDS Control of The Netherlands, Amsterdam.

EL-HAMAD, I., TIRINATO, A., MATTEELLI, A., CASTELLI, F. and CAROSI, G. (1993) 'A health care unit for migrants in Brescia, Italy', in DEUTSCH AIDS-HILFE (Ed.) *Migrants, Ethnic Minorities and AIDS: First European Meeting for the Exchange of Information*, p. 56, Blossin, May.

EUROSTAT (1994) *Census of Population in the Community Countries 1991–93*, Luxembourg: Office de publications officielles des Communautés Européennes.

GATTARI, P., SPIZZICHINO, L., VALENZI, C., ZACCARELLI, M. and REZZA, G. (1992) 'Behavioural patterns and HIV infection among drug-using transvestites practising prostitution in Rome', *AIDS Care*, **4**, pp. 83–7.

GENC, M., AGACFIDAN, A., GERIKALMAZ, O. and MARDH, P.A. (1993) 'A descriptive study on Romanian women prostituting in Istanbul', paper presented at the Third Conference on International Travel Medicine, Paris, Abstract 53.

GERACI, S. (1995) *Argomenti di Medicina Delle Migrazioni*, Busseto, Italy: Ed. Peri Tecnes.

GIULIANI, M. and SULIGOI, B. (1995) 'La sorveglianza epidemiologica delle malattie sessualmente trasmesse negli immigrati', in DA VILLA G. and PASINI, W. (Eds) *Aspetti Sanitari del Fenomeno Immigratorio in Italia*, Rome: Insituto Italiano di Medicina Sociale.

HENDRIKS, A. (1991) *AIDS and Mobility: The Impact of International Mobility on the Spread of HIV and the Need and Possibility for AIDS/HIV Prevention Programmes*, EUR/ICP/ GPA 023, Copenhagen: World Health Organisation.

ISEMAN, M.D. and STARKE, J. (1995) 'Immigration and tuberculosis control', *New England Journal of Medicine*, **332**, pp. 1094–5.

LOUTAN, L. (1992) 'Medical screening of asylum seekers', *International Migration Quarterly Review*, **30**, pp. 223–32.

MARDH, P.A. and GENC, M. (1995) 'Migratory prostitution with emphasis on Europe', *Journal of Travel Medicine*, **2**, pp. 28–32.

OFFICE FÉDÉRAL DES RÉFUGIÉS (1992) *Statistiques en Matière d'Asile 1991*, Berne: Office Fédéral des Réfugiés.

RECTOR, R. (1994) *Migration, Health and AIDS. Supportive Service Needs of Foreigners Affected by HIV: Acceptable, Available and Equitable*, Luxembourg: Final report to the Commission of the European Communities.

SPINACI, S. and ARONSON, B. (1990) 'Towards policy regulations for TB prevention and control in migrant populations', paper presented at the IOM/WHO seminar on migration medicine, Geneva, February, paper No 1.7.

SPIZZICHINO, L. (1993) 'AIDS prevention in the area of male prostitution: Project for male transexuals', in DEUTSCH AIDS-HILFE (Ed.) *Migrants, Ethnic Minorities and AIDS: First European Meeting for the Exchange of Information*, pp. 56–9, Blossin, May.

STARY, A., KOPP, W. and SOLTZ-SZOT, J. (1991) 'Medical health care for Viennese prostitutes', *Sexually Transmitted Diseases*, **18**, pp. 159–65.

SULIGOI, B., GIULIANI, M., BINKIN, N. and THE STD SURVEILLANCE WORKING GROUP (1994) 'The national STD surveillance system in Italy: Results of the first year of activity', *International Journal of STD and AIDS*, **5**, pp. 93–100.

ZURLO, A. and GERACI, S. (1991) 'Social and sanitary framing of migrant phenomenon in Italy', in HAOUR-KNIPE, M. *Assessing AIDS Prevention: Migrants and Travellers Group Final Report*, Lausanne, IUMSP Doc. 72.

Chapter 13

Transnational AIDS/STD Prevention among Migrant Prostitutes in Europe

Licia Brussa

This chapter describes the work of a transnational AIDS/STD prevention project among migrant prostitutes in Europe (TAMPEP). The project combines research and active intervention, promoting awareness on HIV/AIDS and STDs among migrant sex workers. The target groups of our interventions are a varied group of women whom we define, for reasons which will be clarified shortly, as 'migrant prostitutes'.

Prostitution in Europe should be seen as an international phenomenon, involving an increasing number of women and men, from other European countries and from other continents. There has been, since the 1970s, a noticeable influx of persons involved in the sex industry who have migrated from Asia, Africa and Latin America (Brussa, 1991). In addition, and more recently, the industry has seen a constant increase in the number of central and eastern Europeans who have crossed into western Europe, and have been initiated into or continue to practise as sex workers. Interviews performed during the course of TAMPEP activities have made clear that many of the individuals to whom our intervention is targeted had no previous experience of sex work in their country of origin, and had no intention of engaging in this trade when they moved to Europe. It should also be stated that many of those involved in the sex industry do not identify themselves as prostitutes, and think of their work as only temporary.

Both female and transsexual sex workers have been contacted as part of our work. In this chapter, as well as in our work, we respect the gender identification with which transsexual sex workers present themselves to us, and do not consider them a third gender. We refer to transsexuals here as women, since the majority present themselves in this way. They have specific medical and social needs requiring special attention. Such differences are beyond the scope of this discussion, however, and will not be referred to again here.

Prostitution involving migrant sex workers occurs in all countries of the

European Union (EU). Groups are becoming increasingly mobile, both within single Member States and within the larger community. In a phenomenon which merits particular attention, this mobility has activated a structural phenomenon of serial or chain migration, in which an individual who has already found employment in Europe may arrange for friends in the home country to follow. It should be stressed that migrant prostitution is not a temporary or a static phenomenon, and that parallels need to be drawn with the experiences of other groups who migrate to Europe in search of employment.

In many areas within the EU, the number of migrant prostitutes active within the sex industry is greater than that of local sex workers (EUROPAP, 1994). However, migrant sex workers frequently remain outside of legal, social and medical structures, and therefore face enormous difficulties in gaining access to information and resources that could improve their quality of life. This marginalized position also leads to victimization of migrant prostitutes in criminal activities and illegal trafficking of women and men, as well as to isolation and dependency (Brussa, 1994a).

Existing services in the European Union have little contact with members of this target group, and it is for this reason that the TAMPEP project originated in August, 1993, in The Netherlands, Italy and Germany. Austria joined the project in its second phase. The coordination of each of these sites has been the responsibility of the Mr A de Graaf Stichting (Foundation) in The Netherlands, the Comitato per i Diritti Civili delle Prostitute (Committee for the Civil Rights of Prostitutes) in Italy, and Amnesty for Women in Germany, LEFI/Lateinamerikanische Exilierte Frauen in Osterreich in Austria.[1] The objective of the project is to develop, in collaboration with migrant sex workers, more effective strategies to facilitate contact with the target group, as well as new materials. The four organizations involved in the project had already played an active role in the field of prostitution in their respective countries, and functioned as a reference for migrant prostitutes. This previous work in the field determined the philosophy and conduct of the project, and facilitated making contact.

The TAMPEP Project

The creation of TAMPEP was initially motivated by three factors. First, there was the lack of HIV/STD information available in the native languages of the target group. This lack impedes the development of educational and preventive programmes concerning risks linked to the professional activities of the sex workers. In addition, it makes it difficult to improve their working conditions and, consequently, poses an obstacle to opportunities for improving physical or psychological well-being. Second, are issues linked to the living and working conditions of migrant sex workers. Some sex workers live in conditions of great need with regard to health and hygiene. The general conditions prevalent in establishments or venues where migrant prostitutes are professionally active also create such needs. Third, it is important to facilitate direct contact between migrant sex workers and institutions active in the social and medical fields. This contact should allow for cultural mediation while not compromising the delivery of an efficient service.

During its first year of activities, TAMPEP conducted experimental outreach work in very diverse regions. The respective countries and/or regions differ in immigration policies, in the application of laws relating to prostitution, and in the ways in which sex work is organized and practised. The sites also differ in health-care structure, and in the organization and implementation of health promotion activities, especially those targeted towards HIV/STD prevention among sex workers. Finally, activities were conducted with sex workers originating from a very wide range of cultures. It should be clearly stated that the project did not set itself the objective of creating a network of services capable of covering the needs of entire countries.

There are many different forms of prostitution. The forms of the sex business in which migrant prostitutes most often work are in street prostitution, sex clubs, shop windows and private apartments. Each of these has its own specific working conditions, but what they all share is the fact that the population of sex workers is very international, and that the concentration of any specific nationality varies from different host country to country. There were a total of twenty different nationalities among our target group, from Latin America, west Africa, south east Asia, and from eastern Europe and the Balkan countries. Some from among the very many different situations covered by the project, and drawn from the project's field work, are described below.

The Shop Window in The Netherlands

Most of those working in shop windows are migrants, from the Dominican Republic, Colombia, Venezuela, Ghana, Benin, Poland, Russia, the Ukraine, Lithuania, Serbia, Croatia, and the Czech and Slovak Republics. Sex workers pay rent for the windows, about 150 florins (US$ 90) a day, although this varies. The woman waits for clients in a room with a window that looks on to the street. The room contains the bed where she works, and also lives and sleeps. In some establishments two sex workers may share a kitchen, a room for eating, a bathroom and toilet. At some sites the buildings comply with general sanitary and administrative rules for the municipality, security is assured by men patrolling the street, rents are fixed, and neither minors nor victims of trafficking are allowed to work. In others, up to four women may use the same window room, share a single toilet, an improvised shower and no kitchen. In some cases workers receive one towel and two sheets for use throughout the week. On average, the sex workers interviewed work between twelve and seventeen hours a day, receiving from ten to twenty-four clients, at a usual charge of fifty florins for fifteen minutes' work.

Sex Workers from Brazil in Hamburg

Among the sex workers of both sexes and from all continents who work in a variety of sites in Hamburg are Brazilian women and transsexuals. The majority of the women come from the poorest region of Brazil. Many had already worked as sex workers before they arrived: some had been initiated into the business when they were children. Others had believed promises about earning quick and easy money, or hoped for marriage. For many, sex work is the choice of freedom and independence, a way of escaping poverty, family violence, exploitation and loneliness. In Hamburg they work in apartments, bars and clubs. Some support children or family back in Brazil; others are transsexuals who feel they will be more free to live out their identities outside their own country.

Eastern European and Latin American Sex Workers in Italy

Although soliciting and the exploitation of prostitutes by third parties is prohibited by law in Italy, a number of clubs and discotheques engage 'entertainers'. 'Talent agencies' arrange to have women hired as dancers and transferred from club to club every two weeks. When their visas expire after three months, the workers either return to their country of origin or become clandestine. Those engaged in sex work in night clubs, and who are in the country illegally, are vulnerable to exploitation, including trafficking. The official duty of the women working in the clubs is to eat, drink and dance with clients, and they earn a commission on the number of drinks consumed. Anything earned from sexual activity with the clients tends to belong exclusively to the women in question. Women involved in this area of the Italian sex industry come from several regions, including Latin America, south-east Asia and eastern Europe. Relations between prostitutes of different nationalities in the same circuit of sex work are almost non-existent.

TAMPEP field work revealed that in all countries where the project operated, there was a stratified population of migrant sex workers: one distinct category resides in the host country for an extended period (at least five years) and engages at most in internal mobility within the host country, or works for very brief periods in other European countries. A second category is that of transients, who move continually throughout various states, and whose presence in each is always of short duration. There is a difference, then, between sex workers who choose to emigrate more or less permanently to one of the four countries, and who constitute a rather stable group, and those who represent a new flux of trans-European migration. Migrant sex work is characterized by constant changes in the make-up of the target group, with frequent variations in the concentration and number of such workers in any of the four countries participating in the project, in the nationalities represented, and in their degree of mobility.

The variety of policies concerning immigration from outside the European Union, and differences in possibilities for obtaining a residence permit, influence the living and working conditions of migrant sex workers. These differences also increase their marginalization, and facilitate possibilities for exploitation, dependency and control by criminal organizations. In particular, the severity of regulations recently enacted in Europe against non-Europeans directly influences the basic living and working conditions of clandestine migrant sex workers. Those who are clandestine and work in closed prostitution (apartments, window brothels, sex clubs) remain constantly within the same milieu. Since they rarely, if ever, have an opportunity to leave the context of work or of the sex industry, their lifestyle is one of severe isolation and marginalization, with damaging consequences to physical and mental well-being.

Strategies of Approach

The method used by TAMPEP, applied in all four partner states, involves active and direct participation and collaboration with the target groups. Sociological investigation and practical interventions for AIDS prevention were developed in a continuous cycle of gathering information, organizing activities based on the data gathered, creating new materials and evaluating results. Provisional findings from the evaluations were then put into practice in new activities. This continuous process of investigation, production of material, implementation and evaluation has permitted the development of grass-roots activities tailored to each group and subgroup. It has allowed us to work towards positive interventions to improve the health of sex workers.

The concrete activities of the teams have been to conduct interviews to gather general information concerning migrant prostitution in Europe;

to conduct an initial needs assessment with sex workers; to test and adapt existing materials; to develop new materials in collaboration with the target group; to carry out workshops and provide individual consultations; to encourage the development of adequate services by governmental institutions; to mediate, refer and accompany sex workers to service providers; to train peer educators; to continuously evaluate the effects of the activities, focusing on levels of knowledge, attitudes towards health promotion, and behaviour changes in the direction of safer sex and other health behaviours; and to identify structural impediments to achieving the above.

The target group for our project has characteristically been hard to reach. As with other marginalized populations within society, there is an increasing recognition of the influential role of informal peer educators and supporters in facilitating access to information about and for the community. Interventions have thus been developed through the use of these two types of intermediaries, cultural mediators and peer educators.

Cultural Mediation and Public Health Services

> Cultural mediators are a go-between who know the reasons, the customs and the codes of a majority culture and the host country, as well as the conditions, social ethics and the scene in which a minority group finds itself. (Brussa, 1995 p. 78)

Cultural and linguistic mediation can help stimulate new models of intervention. It may also serve as an example for integrating immigrants into a particularly important arena, that of public health services. In their contact between clients and service providers, cultural mediators serve as a bridge, proving the need for raising awareness, and verifying the perceptions of both sides. Their work is with the many factors intervening between a migrant group and those who provide services for international clients. At the same time, they can facilitate contacts with a population seen to be problematic and burdensome.

Cultural mediators are not social workers, health assistants or exclusively translators. In the TAMPEP project they are individuals capable of eliciting the trust of the target group, and of the same ethnic group or nationality as the sex workers, thereby being capable of recognizing and appreciating the cultural and social mechanisms influencing their behaviours and choices. Cultural mediators are also educators and trainers, with a mandate to pass on knowledge and experiences in the field of STD/AIDS prevention among sex workers. They are recognized as such by the target group. Cultural mediators belong to a 'different' culture, interacting with, and reacting to, the dominant culture of the host country. They facilitate communication between members of an immigrant community and those of the dominant culture, as well as with other individuals or groups who in some way have contact with the migrant sex worker. They serve as a point of reference since they, themselves, have had the experience of migration and, in some instances in our case, also experience within the sex industry.

In their work linking migrant sex workers and service providers, cultural mediators seek to explain host country health systems to people whose ideas and experiences with public health services in their own countries may be quite different. They negotiate and illuminate a variety of non-verbal messages in the way in which the clients address themselves to the service providers. They intervene in the many factors which hinder the access of migrant sex workers to health systems. These factors go beyond the obvious problems of language, and include problems related to specific cultures, to the general situation of the migrant sex worker in the host country, to levels of education and to the sexuality of the worker.

Mediators must be able to maintain a position of autonomy, of neutrality. Their responsibilities go far beyond linguistic interpretation: in the course of their work they translate cultural concepts rather than mere words. The role of cultural mediators in the TAMPEP project is thus a very complex one. On one side, mediators may be perceived by sex workers as healers. On the other side, they may be seen as advocates for the services themselves, rather than for the target group. In this case the risk is that cultural and linguistic mediators may be perceived as accomplices of the services, thus in part responsible for behaviours which cause dissatisfaction among the target group. Mediators inevitably find themselves trapped between two blocks: service providers may have unrealistic expectations about the effects of cultural mediation, and sex workers themselves who may nurture unrealistic expectations concerning mediators' possibilities to improve health services. It must be made clear to both parties from the outset that cultural mediators cannot provide guarantees to either party.

Cultural mediation

Merely offering free, anonymous testing or screening does not in itself guarantee access to many of those who most require such services. Just because a door is open does not mean that entry is any easier if one does not know where the door is located, or even that it exists. Just getting in a door does not mean that one necessarily enjoys the room in which one finds oneself. For example, although there are no policies of mandatory STD screening in Hamburg, and no direct control is exercised over prostitution venues to ensure regular medical check-ups, in the minds of many sex workers public health services still connote institutions characterized by repressive measures and attitudes. Many, in addition, have professional experience in other areas of Germany in which mandatory screening is conducted by the municipal health service. It is obvious, therefore, that many migrant sex workers are not in a position to construe visits to the public screening and treatment centre for STDs/HIV as anything but coerced controls conducted with the complicity of pimps. In a situation fraught with ambiguities, *one* of the challenges of cultural mediation is to promote the centre's vision of medical care and check-ups as a tool for health promotion and self-esteem.

Peer Educators

In contrast to cultural mediators, peer educators are members of the target group, and therefore identify themselves completely with the group. They play the role of leaders, and articulate the interest of their peers. The experience of the TAMPEP project with peer education targeted towards a specific group of sex workers (mobile migrants who are frequently marginalized and in a position of dependency) has provided insight into the advantages and limitations of the approach, and as to certain modifications which may need to be introduced in applying concepts of peer education.

Our experience has shown that there are some preconditions for effective peer education. Generally speaking, peer educators must have a base in the community, and must be recognized as leaders by the community base, while being representatives of the particular project being developed. Experience has shown that the success of peer educators depends more on their self-identification with the role, and on their acceptance within the community, than on their specific position within it. Peer educators must also be clear about their role both within the group and within the project. Peer education implies a didactic role, and influencing changes in behaviour. Educators should be able to raise awareness among their colleagues, and to organize and conduct workshops on various themes related to prevention and safer sex practices in the field of AIDS/STDs. Their role implies a certain distancing, which facilitates the assumption of a student–teacher relationship. While they have the role of imparting information and knowledge, increasing responsibility and self-esteem, peer educators must also make distinctions between their community work and their own and other sex workers' private lives (their romantic involvements, professional contacts and career). They must also be able to apply the concept of peer education with a community that is extremely mobile. As opposed to cultural and linguistic mediators, peer educators do not need to have either a relationship of confidentiality or a 'mandate' from the group with whom they identify. Their primary focus is on mutual support among colleagues for sustaining behaviour changes in adopting safer sex.

Training Nigerian Sex Workers in Turin

The creation of a drop-in centre for Nigerian (and other African) sex workers in Turin is a concrete example of how banding together around a common idea and a shared base served to mobilize a community, and to lead to further activities. The group of fifteen active and recently retired sex workers who had participated in the development of the drop-in centre were successively trained and functioned as peer supporters. They collaborated on the development of material, translated and promoted the project's activities. Once this structural base was established, the workers identified twenty additional Nigerian sex workers from five different tribes who, in turn, underwent structured training courses on AIDS, STDs and the female reproductive system. These peer-education courses have been repeated three times, each time with a new group of participants.

Using Mobility

A travel route is formed by a network of contacts among fellow nationals who inform others of work opportunities, with a snowball effect. Other networks are formed by individuals who channel women within a circuit managed by people external to the sex industry. In both cases a sex worker's period of residency within a country may be extremely brief. This form of mobility is inherent to migrant prostitution, and what at first glance may seem as a handicap may be taken as an opportunity. The fact that frequent mobility may limit possibilities for repeated contact with the target group should not detract from the equally valid fact that that said mobility can contribute to a further dissemination of health-promotion messages within the same circuits: it should be possible for those involved to become health messengers. So far the project has been able to use this phenomenon only to a limited extent, but that the possibility exists is demonstrated when sex workers interviewed as a control group, who had not been involved with the project's activities, had already heard of TAMPEP through colleagues encountered in the new workplace or through fellow nationals before they left.

Preliminary Results

Because of the extremely marginal and vulnerable conditions in which migrant prostitutes live in European countries, and through the experience gained during the first year of the project, both by the direct contact with migrant prostitutes and by an assessment of their living conditions, we have concluded that STD and HIV/AIDS prevention for this group must be included in a broader framework of general health promotion. The development of such a framework should be recognized as a present priority.

It has become clear that a number of migrant sex workers in certain areas of The Netherlands, Italy, Austria and Germany are willing to collaborate in the design and implementation of activities of projects such as TAMPEP. We are now working with these individuals. Another important observation is that, although many projects employ strategies and materials designed for 'western' eyes, women from different cultural backgrounds need totally different approaches, strategies and materials.

After three years of the project, we have found that social control and social cohesion are important factors in increasing the capacity of sex workers to challenge clients who are unwilling to practise safer sex. We have thus attempted to boost group cohesion among migrant sex workers in an attempt to positively influence their articulated and implicit codes of conduct. These strategies will improve both the initial bargaining position of the sex workers and their negotiating techniques. We believe that it is necessary to focus on augmenting the self-confidence and, consequently, the self-efficacy of the sex workers. Women must be supported in their efforts to gain control over their working and living conditions. By building on naturally existing contacts, peer leaders and educators have a crucial role to play in this process. A broad spectrum of community-based initiatives directed at empowerment of migrant sex workers can have a major impact on primary prevention in that it allows sex workers increased scope in their negotiations with clients, brothel owners and pimps.

Guidelines

In 1993, a consultant working with the then WHO Global Programme on AIDS, Office of Intervention and Support (IDS) produced draft guidelines to assist countries and organizations in developing methods and prevention projects for safe work for prostitutes (Alexander, 1993). Although this report has never been formally published, TAMPEP and many other organizations throughout the world have benefited from these draft guidelines, and have used them as a political base for their projects. These are as follows:

- Prostitutes should be able to protect themselves from HIV infection, AIDS and other STDs. They should have safe working conditions, including the right to turn down abusive or uncooperative clients, and should have the right to refuse to engage in practices likely to

transmit HIV and other STDs, including any penetrative sex performed without a condom.
- Prevention activities should be targeted to various audiences within the sex work sector: sex workers, clients, lovers and other non-commercial partners, sex work business owners and managers, health-care workers, police . . .
- The practice of safer sex by sex workers is linked to safe working conditions.

It cannot be stressed enough how important the involvement of members of each target group can be in devising strategies to work with this audience. Peer education has been a major strategy in AIDS prevention, and in the most successful projects has led to a strengthening of a sense of community and, among sex workers, professionalism (Alexander, 1992).

Conclusion

It is not only cultural diversity that creates diversity in attitudes: more important is the particular context of the sex industry in which migrant prostitutes are employed; the structural factors regarding prostitution in the host country; and the health policies that have a direct impact on the social and working conditions of subgroups within a targeted population. Moreover, the possibilities for sex workers to have optimal control over their sexual services and the promotion of their health in general, is determined more by the control they have over their working and living conditions, and by their legal status in Europe, than by their cultural and national background. There must be constant collaboration with the sex workers, in which a space is created to allow them to define their own needs and priorities, to create their own materials and activities, and to make their demands within the ambit of European prostitution.

Those who work with migrant sex workers should ideally be of the same nationalities and cultures as the migrant sex workers themselves. This allows effective and direct dialogue, and working group members can function as cultural mediators between the prostitutes and all possible service providers. Partial results, effective implementation of activities, ways of adapting existing materials and methods, and ongoing evaluations need to be periodically reviewed in order to make them as effective as possible.

Leaflet distribution alone is insufficient to bring about behaviour change. The basis of the work must be in continuous and intensive field work to establish trust. Individual and group counselling (including on social, legal and psychological matters) is necessary to facilitate behaviour changes. Supporting migrant sex workers to empower themselves in other aspects, such as in improving working conditions, in the social sphere, and in their legal status, must also be part of any intervention, as this will enable them to control their own lives.

Continuous collaboration with health services is crucial in ensuring that information on safer sexual behaviours reaches migrant sex workers. The role of the programme in this should be focused more specifically towards that of mediating between the sex workers and the medical services, shaping and gaining official backing for cooperative models to be adapted according to local circumstances in each country.

Interventions promoting safer sex practices alone are not sufficient. Informing migrant sex workers about the right brand of condoms, instructing them in proper use, and teaching negotiating skills need to be supplemented by direct field work — actual assistance in going out to buy condoms, or creating the conditions so that they are supplied condoms that are adequate. Similarly, informing sex workers of the value of regular preventive medical attention must be complemented with referral to addresses of empathic doctors. In other words, campaigns to give information and to promote health without connecting these campaigns to service provision will not be effective.

The mobility of migrant sex workers within Europe requires that concepts of 'peer education' be adapted. This mobility can be used in a positive way: when peer educators are trained in the fundamentals of safer sex and health promotion, they can function as 'health messengers' as they move through Europe. Ideally, they should be supported by an international network of intervention projects. On the other hand, the possibilities for non-European prostitutes to create an autonomous organization and to work together in a community-based model focusing on human rights and advocacy, is limited by the legal status of clandestine migrants and by the marginalization to which they are subjected. A further limitation to group work stems from the fact that for the majority of foreign sex workers, prostitution represents a means of survival, an activity practised out of economic necessity. It is seen as temporary work, and in no case as an identity.

The project has developed a number of leaflets, and one might have the impression that now that these have been developed, future work can restrict itself to distributing them among new groups. This would be to miss the most important aspect of the method: the process of making the leaflets is important in itself. Making material stimulates discussions of their needs among the women and men involved, and fosters group cohesion. Thus each activity with a new group should include the production of new leaflets: each particular situation calls for new items, and is in itself a very important educational activity. Moreover, leaflets serve as a written reminder after a working group session or an individual communication, but they cannot function as an information tool in themselves.

It is necessary to establish a network of contacts both within the sex work milieu and within the broader community. Proprietors of prostitution businesses obviously often play a decisive role influencing working and sanitary conditions in their houses, and affecting the possibilities of practising safer sex. TAMPEP has now found that influencing proprietors, with the support of medical and health authorities, is a powerful tool in changing structural circumstances.

The presence of migrant sex workers in the European sex industry constitutes a phenomenon which has changed all aspects of the market. Current European policies in the areas of prostitution, of migration, and of AIDS prevention do not reflect this. The aims of AIDS prevention are often in contradiction with those of migration prevention (to stop the inflow of persons from outside European countries). The effects of these policies are at the moment counter-productive: migrant sex workers are not stopped at the border, but are more and more dependent on, and under the control of, international criminal organizations. This clearly does not serve the interest of either safer sex or of public health.

Note

1   Mr A de Graaf Stichting, Westermarkt 4, 1016 DK Amsterdam, The Netherlands, tel: +31 20/6247147. Coordination: Licia Brussa, Jan Visser.

Comitato per i Diritti Civili delle prostitute, Casalla Postale 67, 33 170 Pordenone, Italy, tel: +39434/57 2901 Coordination: Pia Covre, Carla Corso.

Amnesty for Women, Louse-Schröder-Str. 31, 22767 Hamburg, Germany, tel: +49 40/38 753 Coordination: Veronica Munk.

LEFÖ Lateinamerikanische Exilierte Frauen in Österreich, Kettenbrückengasse 15/4, 1050 Viena, Austria, tel: +43 1/58 11880 Coordination: M.C. Boiles.

TAMPEP has benefited from the financial assistance and support of the Praeventie Fonds (the Dutch Preventive Fund) and the Commission of the European Communities, Directorate General Employment, Industrial Relations and Social Affairs; Health and Safety Directorate, Public Health (DG V).

References

ALEXANDER, P. (1992) 'Some considerations regarding trafficking in women and exploitation of prostitution in relation to HIV/AIDS prevention', paper presented at the Inter-Sessional Working Group of the Commission on the Status of Women, Vienna.

ALEXANDER, P. (1993) 'Making sex safer: A guide to HIV/AIDS interventions', Geneva, WHO Global Programme on AIDS, Office of Intervention and Support, unpublished doctoral dissertation, GUIDTOC:GD4.

BRUSSA, L. (1991) *Survey on Prostitution, Migration and Traffic in Women: History and Current Situation*, Council of Europe, EG/Prost.

BRUSSA, L. (Ed.) (1994a) *TAMPEP: Final Report*, Amsterdam: Mr A. de Graaf Stichting.

BRUSSA, L. (Ed.) (1994b) *TAMPEP: Manual*, Amsterdam: Mr A. de Graaf Stichting.

BRUSSA, L. (Ed.) (1995) *TAMPEP: Analyses the First Year* 1993–4, Amsterdam: Mr A. de Graaf Stichting.

COSPE (1993) 'Cooperazione per lo sviluppo dei paesi emergenti', *Atti del Seminario di Bologna Sulla Mediazione Linguistica e Culturale*, Firenze: COSPE.

EUROPAP (1994) *European Intervention Projects on AIDS Prevention for Prostitutes: Final Report*, EUROPAP, Gent.

NETWORK OF SEX WORK PROJECTS (1994) *European Symposium on Health and the Sex Industry: Final Report*, Edinburgh.

Chapter 14

International Networking:
Building Migrants' Networks across Europe

Petra Narimani, Felix Gallé and Jaime Tovar

> Working and cooperating with different minorities is part of our mutual solidarity. We must always think globally, also when we act regionally. (Extract from the Policy Programme, Grundsatzprogramm IAF, Frankfurt, 1995)

Networking can be highly effective in spreading information, in promoting the exchange of experience and skills between AIDS service organizations (ASOs), and in advocating for the rights of individuals and affected communities, care and support, and the right to live free from discrimination. Since the problems confronted in individual countries are rarely unique or completely new, each can benefit from access to a variety of solutions and programmes: European collaboration can increase the effectiveness of prevention efforts among many different communities. Community-based organizations (CBOs) often serve as the only voice for marginalized groups which have suffered discrimination; this is valid for gay men, commercial sex workers, injecting drug users and for migrants and ethnic minorities, a group that suffers from double or even triple discrimination.

Networking among ASOs and CBOs is a process of self-empowerment, a response to AIDS at local, national and international levels with particular focus on people living with HIV/AIDS and those affected by the disease. It supports newly developed NGOs with limited resources by developing mechanisms for support and exchange of experiences with those better established.

International cooperation is particularly important in the case of migrants who, because of their mobility and often marginal socio-cultural position, have specific needs for AIDS information, care and support. In some European countries, migrant communities have established their own CBOs. In this chapter we will discuss networking among migrant ASOs and CBOs throughout Europe. The advantages and problems of networking are presented in a first, more theoretical, section. In the second part of the chapter, we describe some examples of networking in which the authors have been involved.

What Are the Benefits of Networking?

Harvey (1992) defines a network as 'An international association, union, federation, grouping of organisations, experts or individuals to share information and a common course of action on a problem or issue'. In the broadest sense, the term NGO includes different types and sizes of organizations ranging from small self-help groups to volunteer and large membership organizations. At one end of the spectrum are groups that provide services (counselling, care and support to people with HIV/AIDS and their families). At the other end are groups who seek to influence the broader socio-political and economic environment in which they operate (WHO, 1994).

A major issue for organizations is *policy development*. For migrants in Europe, the Schengen Agreement (allowing free travel for citizens of Spain, Italy, Portugal, Belgium, The Netherlands, Luxembourg and Germany to another Member State) implies that people from countries outside the European Union are subjected to stricter security codes, fuelling feelings of harassment among ethnic minorities and migrants in the name of security and illegal movement. Harmonization of European Union (EU) policies on asylum are planned, but at present there are no established common criteria. There are many disadvantages for migrants living in EU Member States: without EU citizenship they are usually not allowed to vote in their host countries, nor do they have the ability to influence political decisions. Although the largest migrant community in Europe are Turks, their children born in Germany, for example, do not automatically receive a German passport. In Belgium, children whose parents have died before acquiring official status are not allowed to remain in the country after their eighteenth birthday. Effective lobbying by migrant organizations could make things easier by helping people understand their special circumstances, and bringing equal access to social and health services. The European Commission plays an important role in the formulation and development of policies, and a strong CBO/NGO voice could be developed by the appointment of existing networks of migrant organizations and ASOs as observers and delegates on Commission committees or working groups.

While lobbying and political activities within the EU are often confusing, frustrating and time-consuming, and migrant organizations and ASOs always have other urgent needs with which to cope, long-term change is impossible without them. Only powerful networks, united voices from many different groups, can influence policy. The political agenda must be discussed in a broad context, across different groups and across countries. For a variety of reasons, not the least of which are their legal and social disadvantages, it is difficult for migrants to take the initiative of approaching political powers. It is thus even more necessary to strengthen CBO/NGO network capabilities.

Learning how to design a project proposal and a budget in order to gain access to funds are also sound reasons for networking. As budgets are cut it has become increasingly important that organizations know how to present their ideas and what components are currently a priority for funding agencies. Within the network there are organizations with similar problems and project ideas, and common projects have better chances of receiving financial support.

Networks may provide powerful and efficient tools to overcome taboos, feelings of isolation, guilt and disempowerment. The impact here should not be underestimated. To meet others with the same problems, and who understand what one is talking about, can make an individual feel understood and accepted. NGO meetings where information and knowledge can be exchanged provide a unique climate for addressing very personal issues. People can do things they normally do not do: laugh, cry, share their personal stories, in a process of empowerment that leads to many fruitful contributions.

In addition, the *common call for respect of human rights* is one of the most vital reasons for migrants to network:

> Human rights provide the guide for the kind of direction of societal transformation that is needed, because the realisation of human rights and dignity is the societal precondition for health . . . We need to identify which rights are a problem, then act to help ensure respect of these rights. This applies global thinking to local action. (Mann, 1995)

In relation to HIV/AIDS, migrants face racism, discrimination and stigma. Migrants usually do not have equal access to health and social care. Concern has been expressed that migrants are being used to test HIV-related drugs without proper information or even without their consent, and recent reports from Britain suggest that African women seeking ante-natal care have been subjected to HIV testing without their informed consent, identified on the sole basis of coming from a 'high-risk area'. In Germany, there is concern that many asylum seekers and refugees are tested on arrival. Since autumn 1985, all students from developing countries planning to study in Germany under special programmes offered by the Bundeministerium für wirtschaftliche Zusammenarbeit (Ministry of Economic Cooperation) must be tested for HIV as part of a general health check. Those testing HIV positive must return to their home countries immediately. The official argument for the test is:

> It is of special interest for the home countries themselves that only those can benefit from educational programmes which are able to use their knowledge on a long-term basis for the economic and social development of their countries. This precondition is unfortunately not given for those being HIV infected . . . The danger of spreading infection plays a minor role. The important point is that the objectives of such education programmes must not be endangered.

Most of the students, refugees and asylum seekers speak little or no German and often they do not know what a HIV test is. Currently, appropriate pre- and post-counselling is not provided. One example comes from a refugee centre in Saxony (Germany) where a 13-year-old boy from Zambia, after being tested and receiving the news that he was HIV positive, would stay in bed all day and refused to talk to anyone. When asked how he discovered his infection, the answer was simply that all new arrivals at the centre were being tested for HIV.

No country within the European Union has an official policy of mandatory testing, but there are often large differences between practices and official policies. It is important to find as many sources of pressure as possible, as monitoring the human rights situation, with well-documented examples of practices against policy, are very important for developing strategies of action to counter abuses (see working group on human rights, AIDS and Mobility Project, 1994). As the Council of Europe has welcomed the involvement of NGOs, this is a chance for groups to come together and act on an European level.

Sharing information is another reason to network. A variety of European publications and NGO newsletters provide valuable information on the issues surrounding AIDS and migrants. Human-rights violations can be monitored through these reports, and calls for support and appeals published. Through different media it is possible to compare the different approaches followed in specific countries or in different communities. Events can be announced, reports on workshops, meetings and conferences given, contact addresses published, ideas shared and problems stated. Exchanges of information material, posters and videos can be arranged, saving time and money, and helping people feel better in knowing that other groups in other countries share their ideas.

Another important aspect is cooperation between different regions, between countries of northern, southern, central and eastern Europe. European-wide networking activities have had a significant impact at country-level, in particular for the emerging NGOs in central and eastern Europe. Although reported HIV/AIDS rates are still relatively low in this region, there is a risk of increased transmission due to the rapid social and economic changes. At the same time, over 75 per cent of AIDS cases in the European Union are located in only three southern European countries: France, Italy and Spain. Networking among these regions at different stages of the epidemic can assist emerging NGOs to gain official and public recognition and respectability. This, in turn, can influence potential donors. Fund-raising takes a tremendous amount of time and energy. ASOs credibility with donors is enhanced if they are in coordination with others and not working in isolation. In the current climate of cutbacks on AIDS programmes, northern European countries can perhaps learn from southern European countries which have considerable experience surviving on extremely low budgets.

Migration and AIDS are not among the priorities of most governments, and it has been argued that new structures cannot be financed, and that migration and health as a whole are more important than AIDS and migration. The power of networks is needed to convince policy makers of the special role AIDS is playing for migrant communities (Narimani, 1993).

Building up Migrant Networks

Migrant networks face the same problems as other NGO networks. First, there are continuous *local problems* which need to be solved. An example is that most migrants with HIV/AIDS only seek assistance when they become ill, which usually means that the local organization has to react immediately, and is often unable to find satisfactory solutions. In addition, there is increasing competition among and between NGOs for the limited funds available for work on AIDS, and local NGOs may be at a disadvantage in relation to those larger and better established.

Local problems can be time-consuming, frustrating and keep organizations so busy that networking may become an additional burden rather than a support. The structures created by networks usually mean that additional time, resources and energy must be invested in them, with duties increasing as recognition is gained. Migrant organizations are often obliged to struggle for financial support more than other groups in host countries as, in times of budget cuts, government attention to the issue of AIDS and migration is usually extremely limited.

Most organizations have restricted budgets which do not include costs of travel, and many migrants have difficulties obtaining visas. Additionally, it is difficult to find individuals who speak English well enough to be able to exchange experiences. It is quite easy for Turkish groups to discuss their specific needs and the particular problems faced by their own communities, for example, but in international presentations and explanations of cultural approaches — in a foreign language such as English — the essentials are often lost. Most international papers on AIDS are presented in English, thereby ignoring cultural needs simply because such things cannot be expressed in the same manner as in the language of origin.

There are many different target groups within migrant communities.

Learning from each other is a process of emancipation that cannot be seen as a universal value: it is closely connected with social status, with education, origin and personal experiences. Care must thus be taken when discussing networking from a strictly western European perspective to respect, accept and consider the different approaches and values of other countries, and other cultures. In most migrant communities, talking about sexuality and death is taboo. In addition, experts must cover several issues at a time, as migrant communities are extremely heterogeneous in politics or religion, and accessed differently: it is easy to reach Spanish-speaking communities through parties or *fiestas*, while Vietnamese communities more rarely meet for public occasions. Within communities, furthermore, there may be little understanding between various segments: discrimination and prejudice are as common among migrant communities as among other groups.

Different levels of organizational development can be a barrier, as some groups are very well established and equipped while others struggle to survive. Receiving financial support from different agencies entails different funding policies, different types of reports, different deadlines, all of which may well be in a foreign language for the migrant community. Language places an additional barrier in implementing most activities, as the general lack of formal and professional interpreting and translation services not only raises questions of equal access to services and other rights, but also causes mistrust and insecurity.

Networking eventually means competition, and poses problems of representativity. Grass-roots organizations may not agree with the priorities formally or implicitly established by those who have both the international contacts and the skills required to obtain funding. They may feel that funds should be spread more equally or differently. The problem, simply stated, is that it is impossible to include all of the people all of the time, and there is always a danger that a privileged group of individuals takes exclusive leadership. On the one hand, this is of great advantage since the work of international networks often has to rely on individual personalities and relationships. On the other hand, some representatives may lose contact with their own organizations and end up speaking on their own behalf — forgetting that they have a broader mandate to fulfil. From the point of view of those working in a European or an international arena, it is difficult to explain to the grass-roots organization exactly what it is they are doing since the work is intangible, extremely complex and has its own language. A small grass-roots organization will rarely have either a formal position or a line item in its budget for international networking, so such work has to be continuously explained and justified.

Certain individuals must represent the interests of the network to those outside. How will these representatives be identified? They must be well-known, and at the same time recognized as legitimate by the group: networks need to be open to everyone, and be composed of members that actually represent their member groups. Influencing policies is long and tedious, and rarely produces immediately obvious results. For example, if an intervention by an international NGO influences Albania to change its treatment of gay men and remove legal barriers, the impact will have little effect on a migrant organization in Spain. At home, representatives working in the European arena are often seen merely as privileged, being able to travel abroad, working in an international setting. They may receive little support from their own organization, and are often fighting for a specific issue not supported by it. For this reason, international networkers may feel isolated and forced to work on their own.

There are a variety of reasons why some people become well-known and part of the 'privileged' group. It may be by chance that an individual attends the first meeting of an international or European workshop, and continues to participate once he or she is known. Others may be invited on the basis of reputation in a specific field, or have acquired a particular expertise that it is wise to use. Then there are those who can share funds — they sponsor others, financially support a seminar, or have useful contacts with funding agencies. Of all of these the most important is personal contact.

Finally, competition is also observed on an international level when two or more organizations work on the same issue. Although situations are different in each country, this is a potential problem when seeking funds from international bodies such as the European Union. Most organizations wish to cooperate with each other and oppose this type of competition but the funding priorities of donor agencies can cause problems in determining which organization or issue is to be financed. For the most part there is coordination and cooperation among migrant organizations in Europe, but as more organizations seek funding, this potentially could become a serious problem.

Coordination of a Network

Every network needs a formal structure to function, yet must strive to remain as unbureaucratic as possible. A clear purpose must be defined, and the extent of coordination and cooperation. Additional funds will invariably be both needed and not available, so that existing structures should be used as much as possible: the coordinating role should be taken by somebody already doing a similar job. It is important to strengthen contact with other existing networks as well. In the case of migrants, this may be accomplished through participation in various meetings or workshops. During AIDS conferences, for example, representatives of migrants' groups may meet to discuss coordination of activities and common issues. This happened after a meeting on refugees and asylum seekers where a small group met to prepare a round table on migration issues for the International AIDS Conference in Yokohama. In 1995, a preparatory committee was established with the primary responsibility of organizing the Third Information Exchange on AIDS,

Migrants and Ethnic Minorities. This committee is composed of different representatives from different European migrant communities and people working in the field of AIDS and migration.

Questions of Responsibility

Those playing a central role have a mandate to insure that communication flows between the various groups; clarify the specific focus of each community or organization involved; facilitate contracts; identify similarities; keep the door open to all; provide feedback to conferences and meetings; identify donors; and assure that various groups and migrants with HIV/AIDS take part in decision-making processes. Before responsibilities are accepted, a common European approach must be secured and clear targets and goals defined with all activities clearly contributing to needs. Above all, a network and its activities must develop for the benefit of all communities involved.

Inter-cultural Dialogue

Working on issues of AIDS and migration requires close collaboration with the countries of origin. This is extremely important in prevention campaigns developed in both home and host countries. There are, however, within a network, often significant differences between partners from different countries or regions. Although all may share a commitment to human rights, they may differ in their understandings about goals, priorities and strategies. In discussions on human rights, issues of discrimination against women, different religious practices, taboos within certain societies and other profoundly cultural questions may lead to further problems. Migrants living in Europe may have problems with European ideological orientations emphasizing individual approaches, and defending individual liberties, if they come from cultures in which the focus is more on societies and families, and in which there may be a different understanding of illness and death. None of these difficult questions has ever been solved, and NGOs cannot solve them through the fight against AIDS alone.

Integration on an International Level

Migration and AIDS are international issues. Some problems cannot be solved nationally. Solutions may depend on sharing resources among many countries, or on pressure that ASOs joined together can exert. Solidarity throughout Europe, and globally, between ASOs and people affected by HIV/AIDS can provide needed strength. Working internationally represents shared solidarity and a broader fight for human rights, but it also means potential access to financial supporters worldwide, and an ability to influence international gatherings and global strategies and politics. By being part of the global network, the special needs of migrant communities will be included in our common fight against AIDS.

Practical Experiences: How has Networking Functioned across Europe?

Networking among those in the field of migration and AIDS partly started in 1989 in Montreux when a few participants discussed the issue in a workshop at a conference entitled 'Assessing AIDS Prevention'. The AIDS and Mobility Project was one of the first European projects developed (see Chapter 8, this volume). In London, several local organizations (BHAN, BLACKLINERS) offered information and education as well as care and support to their own communities. In 1991, the NAZ Project, an HIV/AIDS service for the south Asian and Muslim communities (see Chapter 7, this volume) led the way in putting the issue on the AIDS agenda, repeatedly pointing out at NGO meetings that migrants and ethnic minorities need specific approaches. When it was established in 1990, the European Council of AIDS Service Organisations (EuroCASO), a forum of AIDS networks, provided migrant groups a column in their newsletter where they could report on their work, projects and meetings, thereby encouraging others to join them or to establish their own groups.

In May 1992, the AIDS and Mobility Project organized a 'Workshop on AIDS Prevention towards the Turkish Population in Europe' which was followed up by a further meeting in Hanover, Germany, in June 1993 (this time organized jointly by the Ethnomedizinisches Zentrum, AIDS Danisma Merkezi in Berlin, and the AIDS and Mobility Project, with financial support from Deutsche AIDS-Hilfe). Some of the Turkish participants also attended 'The First European Conference on HIV/AIDS for the Muslim and South Asian Communities' organized by the NAZ Project (London, September 1992). This event was financially supported by the Commission of the European Communities and the WHO Regional Office for Europe. The initial response was low, but when specific individuals working in the field of migration and/or HIV/AIDS were approached, a large number of potential delegates were identified. This led in Germany, for example, to further networking at the national level, as existing groups were contacted and informed about the goals and targets of the proposed international cooperation. In the end, 131 people from eighteen different countries participated in the conference. The structure of the meeting evolved around a process of individual and group empowerment, and was not based on official representation but on personal experiences and understanding. The conference report served as an important tool for strengthening the network. At the IXth International Conference on AIDS in 1993 in Berlin, round table discussions and satellite meetings provided ethnic minorities and migrant communities the opportunity to discuss the issues of migration and AIDS. Recommendations from previous meetings could be presented and discussed with other people in the field.

In November 1993, The African Foundation for AIDS Prevention and Counselling (AFAPAC) was established in The Netherlands. The need to establish such an organization became evident following research comparing the Ghanaian community in The Netherlands with a cross-section of Ghanaians in Ghana. The study revealed that Ghanaians living in Ghana on average were much more informed about HIV/AIDS than those living abroad. This was initially surprising: people in Ghana believed that Ghanaians in Europe should be well informed about the infection. Currently, AFAPAC targets all Africans who live in The Netherlands and who come from Africa south of the Sahara. The project, closely linked to the AIDS and Mobility Project, participated in the last two European migrants' meetings, and played an important role in organizing the Third European Meeting on Migration and AIDS in The Netherlands in September, 1995.

The First European Workshop on HIV/AIDS in Relation to Refugees and Asylum Seekers organized in 1994 in The Netherlands by the AIDS and Mobility Project brought together thirty experts from fourteen countries. Recommendations, background papers and country reports served as useful tools for dealing with this extremely delicate issue of AIDS and migration. During the meeting it became clear to what extent international collaboration and networking are vital in the global strategy on AIDS.

Prior to the IXth International Conference on AIDS in Berlin, it was felt that the issues surrounding migration and AIDS needed to play a more prominent role in the programmes of such conferences. In order to identify the primary issues for European migrant groups, Deutsche AIDS-Hilfe and Verband der Initiativgruppen in der Ausländerarbeit (a national network of migrants projects in Germany) organized the First European Meeting for the Exchange of Information, co-sponsored by EUROCASO. Over fifty people representing thirty organizations from fourteen European countries participated in the first exchange meeting in Blossin in 1993. As described by the WHO/EURO representative, meetings of this kind represent:

> ... a significant step forward in terms of breaking the vicious spiral evolving from increasing levels of HIV transmission in migrant and ethnic minority communities, increasing racism, scapegoating and 'witchhunting' from the outside world, and the understandable, yet

unfortunate reaction of these communities in terms of reinforce-
ment of denial, taboos and complacency. (Mikkelsen, 1993, p. 32)

The initial idea had been partly self-centred, to learn about different approaches and experiences from other European initiatives in order to establish a project run by migrants in Berlin, since existing organizations had
been unable to meet the needs of migrants in relation to AIDS (indeed the
establishment of AKAM, the AIDS coordination and referral centre for migrants, described below, was a direct result of this meeting). Invitations were
sent to a broad and non-specific list of projects, groups and individuals with
experience in the fields of migrants, ethnic minorities and AIDS, as well as
to those already actively working in these areas.

The aim of the meeting was not to come to decisions based on origins,
culture or religion, but to bring together groups of migrants who, until then,
had limited experience in this type of meeting or with networking. The first
meeting tried to be as heterogeneous as possible, to develop an informal
connection between the participants which would yield the benefits of working together without loosing the autonomy of independent projects. There
was no attempt to establish a unique working model but, rather, possibilities
which would be flexible and adaptable to specific needs while strengthening
the commitment and knowledge of all participants. Workshops and oral
presentations covered a wide range of topics and issues. Issues such as racism, problems with legal rights to remain in Europe, continuity of care for
people who move from country to country while living with HIV, the closing
of borders in 'Fortress Europe', access to medical care, and the right to prevention information in the languages appropriate and relevant to migrant
groups.

One conclusion drawn from the meting was to encourage the establishment of projects in the field of AIDS prevention and assistance for the migrant population in every country. Those responsible for these activities were
to be governments of the host countries and their ministries of health and
education; global and European organizations such as the WHO and the EU;
governmental and non-governmental organizations working in the AIDS field;
migrant organizations and associations including churches, trade unions and
employers' organizations. The working groups prepared several letters to
these organizations and institutions agreed upon by the participants. These
model letters, published in November 1993 as part of the meeting documentation, were also sent to the host countries of the different participants.

The conference report was published immediately afterwards, and presented at the Berlin International AIDS Conference in June 1993 (DAH, 1993).
Another result of the meeting was the establishment of a working group to
continue developing cooperation and strategies of intervention and prevention, and to organize follow-up meetings. Many of the participants have
remained in contact with one another, enabling groups to access information, materials and advice concerning translations of materials and models of

good practice, as well as support over human rights' violations. An active grass-roots network has developed.

The Second European Information Exchange Meeting on Migrants, Ethnic Minorities and AIDS was held in June 1994 at Alden Biesen, Belgium, bringing together sixty participants from organizations in Europe (AIDS and Mobility Project, 1995). The theme was human-rights, with particular focus on how community-based organizations, with their limited funds and resources, could be better informed and equipped to deal with human-rights abuses. There was also felt to be a need to build better links with international human-rights organizations. The objectives of this second meeting of the network were to develop a coordinated approach to lobbying and advocacy on the issues of Migrants and HIV/AIDS in Europe; develop networking in order to work more efficiently together at a European level and to avoid duplication; develop practical methods of assisting community-based organizations with human rights; define ways of influencing policy makers and politicians at national, European and international levels; and provide input into the Yokohama AIDS Conference on the subject of HIV/AIDS and migration in Europe (Tovar, 1994).

A number of recommendations and practical developments emerged, including a call for clear and practical work around both the documenting of abuses of human rights, and developing funding applications. The theme for the next meeting, held in 1995 in Driebergen, The Netherlands, thus became 'skills building'. Less formally, the meeting was also an important opportunity for many of the participants to step back, to reflect on the ways in which their work is carried out, and the many issues held in common.

Developing a Migrants' AIDS-project in Berlin: AKAM

Founded in 1993, AIDS Koordinierungs und Anlaufstelle für MigrantInnen (AKAM) is a community-based organization, offering support to migrants living with HIV/AIDS and fighting discrimination and rejection. At the same time, AKAM works towards the prevention of HIV/AIDS among migrant populations in Berlin. It is grounded in the German National AIDS strategy which rejects control and containment policies in favour of a social education model (Rosenbrock and Salmen, 1990). The formation of a network of self-help groups (Deutsche AIDS-Hilfe e.V. — DAH) has contributed to the formulation of this tolerant AIDS policy: in a unique division of tasks between government and non-governmental organizations (Frankenberg, 1994), the former (represented by Bundeszentrale für gesundheitliche Aufklärung in Cologne) has taken responsibility for public campaigns with the general population, and charged DAH with prevention work within the so-called 'mainly affected groups'. Most local AIDS self-help groups were founded by gay activists, but from the beginning local AIDS-help groups have attempted to integrate other groups as well, such as drug users, prisoners and sex workers (Majer, 1987; Pieper, 1993). The so-called rainbow-coalition was created.

The services AKAM currently provides are information on existing support and care services in Berlin, self-help groups for HIV-positive migrants, support for migrants with HIV/AIDS (translation, buddying, assistance with applications to the German social system). The main target groups for primary prevention are the Berlin Vietnamese, Polish and Hispanic migrant communities. The organization offers a telephone hotline and individual counselling on HIV/AIDS, training for migrant peer educators on HIV/AIDS, educational activities, and the adaptation and production of specific HIV/AIDS information material in different languages.

AKAM has several roots: it is part of the network Verband der Initiativgruppen in der Ausländerarbeit, a local federation of migrant community-based groups. Politically interesting is that with the creation of AKAM a migrants' network has, for the first time in Germany, engaged in the AIDS issue. Several seminars, developed in cooperation with DAH in 1991 and 1992, have led to raising the consciousness of the federation's membership. It was out of a working group on AIDS and migrants that the initiative (described above) came for the First European Information Exchange Meeting, and the proposal to create its own migrants AIDS project (Fonseca, 1991). Migrant communities were no longer satisfied with the services provided by the public health system, and thus took their health and social matters into their own hands (Korporal, 1995).

AKAM would not have been created without the involvement of migrants living with HIV/AIDS. As more and more migrants became infected with HIV and/or fell ill with AIDS, they tried to access existing AIDS-help organizations for services, but the latter are ill-equipped to meet their specific needs (AKAM, 1995). A strategic goal of AKAM has therefore been to involve organizations of migrants in the AIDS issue, and ASOs in the migrants' issue. Since issues of support and prevention for migrants have never been adequately addressed in Germany, AKAM is nurturing a close personal relationship with the self-help potential of DAH. The European network of migrant AIDS organizations provided the impetus to learn from other projects and to clarify priorities.

Conclusion

Networking is important for migrant communities at local, national and international levels. Information and experience can be exchanged and offers of support made. Activities and services can be discussed, coordinated and shared, and matched with skills, resources, needs and target groups. In the long run this process can save manpower, finances and time.

Networking in the field of HIV/AIDS is important to raise awareness about the specific needs of migrant communities, and is essential in efforts to reduce HIV transmission. Some problems have no solutions at the national level: solutions may depend on the shared responses of many communities, or on the combined pressure that groups can exert together.

Networking allows smaller projects to extend their range of influence to the broader political and economic levels, and to advocate, both nationally and internationally, for the rights of individuals and communities affected by HIV/AIDS. Basic needs can thereby be identified and met more effectively. At the same time, international networking is impossible without a solid local basis.

Networking can also serve as a resource of information and expertise for European and international bodies in identifying common needs so as to influence the actions of governments, other NGOs, and international organizations, as well as to urge changes in policies. This is particularly the case in issues too sensitive for a strictly national approach.

Networks, however, are made up of individuals, each with their own very personal story. They are comprised of human beings, with sympathies and antipathies, which means that being part of a network is closely related to the personalities of its representatives. One of the great benefits of networking is being afforded the chance to step back and to reflect on one's work and on common issues. The process of networking is thus empowering, both for the individual and for the community.

References

AIDS AND MOBILITY PROJECT (1994) *First European Workshop on HIV/AIDS in Relation to Refugees and Asylum Seekers*, 29 June–2 July, 1994, Noordwijkerhout, The Netherlands.

AIDS AND MOBILITY PROJECT (1995) *Ethnic Minorities, Migrants and AIDS, Focus on Human Rights and AIDS*, Report of the Second European Meeting for the Exchange of Information, Alden Biesen, June 2–5 1994, Utrecht.

AKAM (1995) *Die Spezifischen Bedürfnisse von MigrantInnen mit HIV/AIDS*, Berlin, AIDS-Koordinierungs und Anlaufstelle für MigrantInnen.

DEUTSCHE AIDS-HILFE E.V. (Ed.) (1993) *Migrants, Ethnic Minorities and AIDS, First European Meeting for the Exchange of Information*, Blossin, 7–10 May, 1993, Frankfurt am Main: Archiv für Sozialpolitik.

EUROPEAN COUNCIL OF AIDS SERVICE ORGANISATIONS (1994) EuroCASO Newsletter, 1/94.

FINK, A. (1993) 'Hier habe ich wenigstens eine Wahl', *Deutsche AIDS-Hilfe Aktuell*, Berlin, Juni, p. 54 f.

FONSECA, R. (1991) 'Im Plural', *Deutsche AIDS-Hilfe Aktuell*, Berlin, December, p. 55.

FRANKENBERG, G. (1994) 'Deutschland: Der verlegene Triumph des Pragmatismus', in

KIRP, D. and BAYER, R. (Eds) *Strategien gegen Aids: Ein Internationaler Politikvergleich*, pp. 134–172, Berlin: Ergebnisse sozialwissenschaftlicher Aids-Forschung, Band 14.

GRUNDSATZPROGRAMM IAF (1995) *Verband Binationaler Familien und Partnerschaften*, Frankfurt.

HARVEY, B. (1992) *Networking in Europe: A Guide to European Voluntary Organisations*, London: NCUO Publications.

KORPORAL, J. (1995) 'Aspekte der psychiatrischen und psychosozialen Versorgung von Migranten', in WIAD SCIENTIFIC INSTITUTE OF THE GERMAN MEDICAL ASSOCIATION (Ed.) *First International Symposium, Migration and Health*, 28 January 1994, **6**, pp. 38–54, Bonn: WIAD Series.

MAJER, S. (1987) 'Möglichkeiten und Probleme der AIDS-Hilfen', in JÄGER, H. (Ed.) *AIDS Psychosoziale Betreuung von AIDS und AIDS Vorfeldpatienten*, pp. 238–52, Stuttgart: G. Thieme.

MANN, J. (1995) *The Next Step: AIDS, Communities and Human Rights*, presented 24 May 1995, François-Xavier Bagnoud Center for Health and Human Rights, Boston, MA.

MIKKELSEN, H. (1993) 'WHO: Global programme on AIDS', in DEUTSCHE AIDS-HILFE (Ed.) *Migrants, Ethnic Minorities and AIDS, First European Meeting for the Exchange of Information*, Blossin, 7–10 May, Frankfurt am Main: Archiv für Sozialpolitik, pp. 32–3.

NARIMANI, P. (1993) 'Non-governmental organisations in Europe: Networking as a tool for information, education and prevention', *Aspects of AIDS and AIDS-Hilfe in Germany*, Berlin: AIDS-Forum DAH, Band XII.

NAZ PROJECT (1992) *Challenge and Response*, The First European Conference on HIV/AIDS for the Muslim and South Asian Communities, London, 9–11 September, London: NAZ Publications.

PIEPER, K. (1993) 'On the history of the AIDS-Hilfe', *Aspects of AIDS and AIDS-Hilfe in Germany*, Berlin: AIDS-Forum DAH, Band XII.

ROSENBROCK, R. and SALMEN, A. (Eds) (1990) *AIDS-Prävention*, Berlin: Ergebnisse sozialwissenschaftlicher AIDS-Forschung, Band 1.

TOVAR, J. (1994) Presentation at Round Table 28, International Conference on AIDS, Yokohama, August 1994.

WHO (1994) *Guidelines for National AIDS Programmes*, Geneva: WHO, Global Programme on AIDS.

Chapter 15

Programme Evaluation

Mary Haour-Knipe and Oonagh O'Brien

The great tragedy of science is the slaying of a beautiful hypothesis by an ugly fact. (Thomas Huxley quoted by Chelimsky, 1994)

Evaluation is an essential component of health programmes in the 1990s, including those concerning HIV and AIDS. The process of evaluation, however, can be fraught with differences of opinion, with struggles over finance, power and influence, so that it comes to be seen as a series of problems, rather than a method of ensuring efficient and appropriate services. Many of the chapters in this book refer to the particular problems arising in trying to meet prevention and care needs around HIV and AIDS for migrants and minority ethnic communities.[1,2] All of these difficulties and problems can be exacerbated if HIV/AIDS interventions are not carefully planned and evaluated at each stage. Good evaluation becomes an essential component if the intervention is to be useful, or even to prevent it from being harmful.

In this chapter we will be discussing evaluation as it specifically concerns HIV/AIDS prevention and care programmes for migrants and ethnic minorities. Just as there is no 'magic bullet' for curing AIDS, there is also no magic bullet for ensuring 'good evaluation' (see Aggleton *et al.*, 1992a; 1992b for more general references on the evaluation of HIV/AIDS programmes). Different approaches will be examined, and we will focus on points particularly applicable to ethnic minorities and migrants. The chapter first reviews the reasons that make evaluation an essential part of a programme, paying attention to needs' assessment, process evaluation, and outcome evaluations for migrant and minority ethnic populations. We then discuss evaluation problems uniquely concerning these target populations. Where relevant, evaluation literature and examples from the authors' own work are introduced. We conclude with recommendations for such evaluations. Both authors have been doing evaluation in this field for several years. One works within the programme in which she has been performing evaluations (Positively Irish Action on AIDS, described in Chapter 7, this volume; O'Brien, 1993; Riordan,

1994; Farrell and O'Brien, 1995; O'Brien, 1995a, 1995b, 1995c), and the other outside the programmes she has been evaluating (the Swiss AIDS prevention programme for migrants, described in Chapter 9, this volume; Fleury *et al.*, 1991; Haour-Knipe *et al.*, 1992; Fleury and Haour-Knipe, 1993; Haour-Knipe *et al.*, 1995; Haour-Knipe and Fleury, 1996).

Evaluation: Why and How

The first reason evaluation is especially important is that the field of HIV/AIDS prevention and care programmes for migrants and ethnic minorities is a new one. Only a few published articles in the mainstream literature deal with evaluation among such populations, and although the number of presentations at international AIDS conferences concerning migrants has been gradually increasing, the quality of such work is extremely variable.[3] The field is also one that is rapidly changing, as several of the chapters in this book attest, and they also reflect the first reason evaluation is important: to describe *how* the programme is doing *what* it is doing (Aggleton *et al.*, 1992b). In a new field we are all to some extent, to put it very simply, inventing as we go along, and good programme description can create transferable knowledge. Good process and outcome evaluation allow a comparison of what works well and what works less well, permitting us to then discuss why an approach may or may not be successful, avoiding needless repetition and waste. A striking example (and also a rare example of publication about a programme that has caused a great deal of trouble) is that analysed by programme evaluators in Israel: in 1991 some 19 000 immigrants arrived from Ethiopia. All over the age of nine were screened for HIV, the decision having apparently been based on the traditional medical and public health approach to infectious disease, without thinking through the differences between HIV and other diseases such as malaria, tuberculosis or hepatitis B, let alone the social consequences. The resulting difficulties were massive: explaining what was going on to the immigrants involved, especially since counselling had not been provided: logistical difficulties in tracing those who were HIV positive, and difficulties providing care to those who followed; breaches of confidentiality; the shunning of people rumoured or known to be HIV positive; the stigmatization of Ethiopians by other Israelis. A frank description of the lessons learned can help others avoid making similar unfortunate choices (Shtarkshall and Davidson, 1995).

Another reason evaluation is important is that preliminary assessment of needs and of the possible best approaches before a programme is designed and implemented can help prevent costly mistakes. There can be no 'ethnic manual' defining once and for all the needs and beliefs of people from a particular culture — as though they were free of influence from the context in which they live — but assessment of community members' ideas concerning the various highly personal realms that need to be discussed where HIV and AIDS are concerned can help prevent needless confusion and distress. Such evaluations can prevent a new programme from blundering in the beginning, marching into the field in inappropriate and possibly harmful ways. Belgian AIDS prevention efforts with the African community, for example (see Chapter 10, this volume), began in 1988 with discussions with community members. Such discussions permitted field workers to learn about such things as ideas about condoms but also, and more importantly, to defuse a climate of suspicion and hostility that had built up surrounding press speculation about the African origin of AIDS.

Baseline evaluation before a programme is established makes it possible to measure change later. We can have some idea of the impact of the Swiss AIDS prevention programme for the Spanish and Portuguese communities, for example, since the AIDS knowledge and condom use were measured among segments of the target population both the year before the programme began and five years later. We will return later in this chapter to the special problems raised, by, before, and after measurements, among migrant populations.

Process evaluation deals with what, why and how interventions or services are delivered, describing what is going on, how the programme is perceived and received, and the group dynamics. Process evaluation will allow those who are running programmes to improve them, to identify problems, bottlenecks, and the first consequences of actions, including those perhaps unintended. Competently done, it also provides field workers an opportunity for critical assessment of their own work, thus encouraging personal and professional development. For example, at Positively Irish Action on AIDS (PIAA) process evaluation allowed the service users to feed back opinions on the organization's service delivery. The agency focuses on helping Irish people with HIV to develop and manage their own care through appropriate agencies. Process evaluation picked up on the fact that some service users did not understand why there was a great deal of input from PIAA when they first made contact, but that contact was reduced when staff felt that individuals were well-equipped to negotiate their own care packages. Once the misunderstanding was identified, more care could be taken to ensure that people understood this process and felt able to return to the agency if their circumstances changed. This has resulted in more satisfaction from service users, and has made it easier to work with a high turnover of people using the service.

Finally, outcome (or impact) evaluation, assessing the effectiveness of the intervention in changing specific outcomes, increases a programme's legitimacy. This effect operates at all levels. By justifying the necessity for a programme, and enhancing its accountability, such evaluation increases credibility towards funders. It may be (and should be) required to substantiate requests for further funding, demonstrating that the programme is going beyond an expression of good intentions to actually achieve something. When an AIDS prevention programme for people seeking asylum, for example, took far longer to put into place than had been anticipated, the external evaluators' discussion of the various problems and resistances raised could support a request for an extra year of funding (Haour-Knipe *et al.*, 1995). When such evaluation is of quality, moreover, and not mere lip service, it can keep institutions honest by dint of its mere presence. Just knowing that an independent evaluation is coming, or can be invoked at any time, can make policy makers, and those running programmes, more prudent and modest in their claims for new programmes, more careful in their accountability, more cost-conscious (Chelimsky, 1994). We return later to problems of causality inherent in outcome evaluation.

Problems and Particularities when Evaluation Concerns Migrant and Minority Ethnic Populations

Methodological problems are, of course, not necessarily specific to evaluating interventions or programmes for migrants. Funding is rarely, if ever, adequate, for programmes, or for evaluations, and both often find themselves simply managing the best they can with what they have. Nor are problems of interdisciplinary work unique to this particular field: health educators, sociologists, anthropologists, psychologists, teachers, physicians, nurses, social workers — the list of different viewpoints is long. Programme goals are too often inadequately specified: they may be fuzzy, or programmes set up with much good will but in a crisis situation may not have been adequately thought through (see Thomas and Morgan, 1991, on American programmes). Or evaluators, target population, and field workers may not share the same clear understanding of the researcher's mandate (see McEwan and Bhopal, 1992, for a discussion). Unpredictability, too, can be considered one of the hallmarks of this field. A well-functioning programme can shift considerably in the light of conditions encountered in the field, focusing on a fortuitous event to make a point, arranging a series of interventions around the availability and interests of a particularly talented volunteer or staff member, or even sending activities off in an entirely new direction when a new problem arises, for example when a community comes face-to-face with a previously denied drug problem as a leader is arrested or a young person dies from a drug overdose. Clear, clean, well-laid-out research designs will more than likely need to be changed, or are in danger of missing the point entirely if they are stuck to. We now turn to methodological problems specific to evaluation with migrant populations, starting with the most obvious.

Gaining Access

All of the problems of talking about stigmatized conditions (HIV and AIDS) with an often stigmatized group (migrants) (see Chapters 6 and 7, this volume) become inflated when there is talk about 'research' among such populations. Both 'research' and 'evaluation' are words that may cause fear, and there is real danger of alienating the target population and thus of harming a programme with a naive or clumsy needs' assessment. Migrants are not necessarily used to academics, or 'the government' taking an interest in them: they may well be suspicious, and justifiably so, of people 'doing research' on them, and AIDS is a poor place for such institutions to start taking an interest in such groups. Communities may feel resentful that nobody shows interest in other issues they perceive as being much more important, such as legal problems, racial harassment, unemployment and housing problems. They may have difficulty distinguishing between those who are working for the programme, and those carrying out the evaluation, or not understand why people are asking the questions they are asking.

Gaining access and trust of the target population can thus involve a long, slow process. Outside evaluators have to prove their legitimacy, their good intentions with the communities, and this puts needs' assessment, especially, into a paradoxical situation in which the assessment should be done before a programme begins, but may not be able to be done until the researchers have demonstrated to the community that they can be trusted, by working with the programme. Even far into programme activities, precautions may need to be taken to avoid misunderstandings. In the latest Swiss evaluation, for example, before a questionnaire was distributed to assess an increase in awareness about AIDS issues among Spanish, Portuguese and Turkish residents in the country, articles were published in the local press of the communities being studied, explaining why the study was being done, how, and what precautions were being taken to maintain confidentiality.

Problems gaining access may also (or perhaps even especially) come not so much from the target population but from the gate keepers who relate to them, including health-care professionals, community leaders, employers and union officials, and social services personnel. Two examples from Switzerland concern authorities responsible for barracks where seasonal workers lived, and those working with asylum seekers: in both cases it was the authorities' wish to protect the people with whom they were working from attention they imagined might be stigmatizing that had to be overcome before evaluators could ask migrants questions related to AIDS.

Working with People of a Different Culture and Language

At a very first level, evaluators need to be sensitive to concerns about racism and stigma. A group's concerns about racism, and/or about labelling, need to be discussed openly before evaluation commences, and concerns arising during it are incorporated into the evaluation process. Similarly, evaluators must be sensitive to gender issues, for example in language, in activities (such as participating in interviews), and in the community-representation roles thought to be appropriate. Second, if materials have to be culturally acceptable, so do the evaluation questions asked. Evaluators are dependent on cultural informants, and getting to know and be able to work with cultural informants also takes time and experience. Field work is essential to thoroughly test interview guides, questionnaires and the like, in order to assure that items are acceptable and understood. In case of doubt detailed information may have to be sacrificed for cultural and political acceptability: in a Swiss study concerning people researchers did not want to risk offending: for instance, we refrained from asking about lifetime number of sexual partners, and simply asked if the respondent had ever had more than one partner.

Related is the problem of language. It is possible, if not likely, that migrants will not be able to speak the language of the host country, or the researcher will not be able to speak the same language as the migrants. It is in any case preferable to interview about sensitive topics in the migrant's own language, but doing so creates added costs and takes extra time. Interviews can be carried out either using interpreters, which means losing direct contact with the interviewee, or by interviewers trained from the migrant group itself. In both cases great sensitivity is required, in choosing an appropriate interviewer, about his or her relationship with the rest of the group, and about maintaining confidentiality within the community.

If a questionnaire is used, it must be translated, then back-translated into the language in which it was originally written to check the accuracy of the translation. Difficulties in translation should not be underestimated. Readers will hardly need to be reminded to what extent AIDS language is a highly specialized one: understandable, but acceptable, terms must be found for issues not ordinarily talked about except in ways that non-specialists would consider vulgar, and the correct term is often the fruit of a long process of testing. Field workers who master the language used in discussions about HIV and AIDS may not necessarily be good translators, and may not be interested in becoming so, and professional translators are not necessarily competent in AIDS language. In addition, the contortions to which researchers resort to maintain ethical neutrality may not necessarily translate very well: a recent Turkish–French back-translation of a questionnaire item on 'transitory sexual relations' or 'casual relations' (not such a simple term in English either) came back translated as 'illicit relations', and tracing the error required lengthy discussions with both translators.

An additional language-related problem is that simple details such as making appointments, or tracing missing documents, become difficult, requiring complicated logistics to make sure somebody is around to do the talking when the telephone rings. Finally, some migrant subgroups may not be able to read any language, rendering distinctly aleatory the use of such quantitative approaches as self-administered questionnaires.

Studying Mobile Populations

Migrant groups are, by definition, highly mobile, and so are many people from minority ethnic groups. An intervention directed towards one group or population will constantly have to be repeated as new people arrive. Long-term evaluation of impact may become impossible if those reached by a programme move on by the time an evaluation can take place, as in the case of asylum seekers, for example, who may stay in a country for months at most. In addition, the target population is often extremely complex. Clandestine migrants are hidden from official statistics (see Watters and Biernacki, 1989), and the size and exact characteristics of even the population legally in the country may be unknown, as official statistics rarely keep up with the movements of such populations. In addition, different waves of migration of people from the same country are liable to be comprised of people with quite different backgrounds, reasons for migrating, and hopes and intentions in the new country.

Typical problems for the impact evaluation of HIV/AIDS programmes are those of multiple influences and of causality: many other things besides the programme being evaluated affect what people know, feel and do about HIV. Such influences in the case of migrants include information from the country of origin which can be acquired before the migrant left, during a holiday visit home, or brought along by a visitor. The evaluation can rarely know quite which influence it may be tapping, and comparison evaluations are difficult, if not impossible. Achieving the 'gold standard' of randomized control trials (Fullerton *et al.*, 1995) is difficult to imagine when working with ethnic minority communities: there is rarely any way of assessing with any accuracy the extent to which differences may be due to the effects of a specific HIV/AIDS programme, or to something entirely different.

Furthermore, some types of programme activity may be difficult to evaluate. In a care and support programme for people who are HIV positive, for example, evaluation may involve assessing quality of life. How do we measure the impact of a counselling session on a bereaved mother? How do we evaluate help with a benefit claim of a recently diagnosed young gay man whose ethnic group does not recognize or allow his sexuality? How do we measure how much difference it may make for an HIV positive Ugandan to have a counsellor from Uganda at the time of diagnosis, rather than a European counsellor, or for someone to have access to appropriate spiritual support at a time of illness? We can never compare such an individual with a 'control' group. We may not even be able to return to ask about the impact of an intervention: in one PIAA study 19 per cent of the respondents were homeless at the time of interview, living on the streets, or sleeping on floors at houses of friends, and 32 per cent had been in this situation at some time in their lives. Evaluating an intervention with persons of no fixed abode in a big city is extremely difficult: one may not be able to find them again.

Different Points of View: Being Inside and Being Outside of the Programme Being Evaluated

Evaluation performed by people from outside a programme may create more *de facto* credibility than evaluation performed by people working within it does, but on several conditions: Chelimsky (1994) points out that it is almost as important for evaluators to understand their user, and thereby be able to explain their findings in terms that make sense to him or her, as it is for the findings to be methodologically strong and compelling in their own right. For evaluation in general, evaluators must first fully understand the programme's objectives and constraints. Second, they must understand the specificity of HIV/AIDS work. And, third, in the case that interests us here, they must in addition be sensitive to the culture of target population(s). Such a mixture of specialized bodies of knowledge is rare.

Evaluation performed by researchers working from within a programme, by personnel linked and committed to it, means that the evaluator is more likely to thoroughly understand the user, and will also play a different kind of role for the organization than an external evaluator. Different questions may be asked. At PIAA the impulse for a research component in the project came from within the community base itself. This is essentially different from partnership, and leads to the community setting their own agenda around evaluation, with the evaluator being seen as fully accountable to the community. The evaluator thereby becomes closely identified with the organization (although this can also happen with external evaluators) and, with a community-based organization, can almost come to play the role of an advocate.

Tensions between Programme and Evaluation

Whether evaluation is performed from the outside or from the inside, tensions between it and the programme are inevitable (see also a discussion by

Power *et al.*, 1991 on relations between evaluation and programme). Evaluation makes many people think of school and of grades, and of somebody telling them whether or not they are doing a good job. In addition, many AIDS/HIV programmes for ethnic minorities and migrants were established in response to a sense of crisis, dealing with a complex and fast-changing health issue under conditions which are very often stressful and emotionally demanding. Such conditions exacerbate the natural tensions between the programme and the evaluation.

Programme staff and evaluators may not thoroughly understand the constraints under which each other is operating: the relationship needs to be clearly negotiated from the beginning, and renegotiated as necessary as it proceeds. Evaluation takes time, time from the programme, and may be indeed difficult for field workers, involved in urgent and real problems, to embrace. They may well feel less time should be spent on paperwork, when friends are dying. For others, filling out a form about an intervention is the last thing they want to do after an evening discussing AIDS and HIV. Evaluators may make supplementary demands on some of the programme's key people, by wanting to interview them, requesting their help with distributing a questionnaire, and so on. Programme staff may feel evaluators are adding strains that may damage their relationships with such personnel, or overburden them, even to the point of risking driving them away from their HIV work. Evaluators' methodological concerns may be perceived as nit-picking, and evaluation and funder-imposed deadlines may not fit in with work loads in the field. One of the authors of this paper, for example, at one time caused considerable animosity by going into the field with a questionnaire just as many of the potential respondents were preparing to leave for their summer holidays.

When evaluators come from outside the programme, time must be spent to make them aware of what is going on in the programme, to assure that methods used in the evaluation are appropriate. When the evaluators work within it, tension can arise when problems, or shortcomings, identified as such by a researcher are not felt to be so by the rest of the team. Close identification with the programme can affect discussions about it, and also the way decisions are made. Evaluators closely identified with programmes may adopt very high standards, finding it hard to praise the programme, pressing for further development and changes, putting pressure on the whole organization; or they may, on the other hand, continuously find excuses for weaknesses.

Finally, evaluation may find itself in a decidedly unpleasant situation if findings are negative. Whether the evaluation is internal or external, it may well be difficult to openly discuss negative findings between evaluators and a project team. The latter may feel unfairly represented and misunderstood. The former may have difficulty finalizing an evaluation when the results are negative, and they feel obliged to be very critical, especially if findings may lead to a programme being cut. There is a momentum to keep programmes going, even if the need no longer exists, and few people like to be even indirectly responsible for colleagues losing their jobs.

Power Differences

Many of these tensions can be attributed to differences in power between the evaluated and the evaluator. Evaluation is often a requirement of funding. AIDS services organizations frequently do not perceive evaluation as 'owned' by the project, but as an external event with which they are forced to comply. They feel they have to 'jump through the hoop' to obtain the required funds to get on with their 'real work', which is to help people with AIDS (see Riordan, 1994, p. 39). Another basis for such differences is that the people carrying out the evaluation and those being evaluated frequently use different spoken and written languages. Evaluators often use academic language, in line with that of funders and health authorities, and have more access to platforms in which to present their opinions. AIDS service organizations do not often have access to the same platforms so as to be able to redress an impression given by an evaluation with which they are not in agreement. Such differences are even more marked when community-based organizations involve minority ethnic groups and migrants. Finally, consultation is often not genuine. It too frequently consists of asking about the acceptability of an already established set of ideas, thus leaving the consulted only the opportunity to be reactive. This is especially the case when ongoing frontline work takes up a great deal of time and energy, making it difficult to switch rapidly into thought processes required to adequately critique proposals.

Methods and Approaches

The key words in discussing methods to overcome these problems are sensitivity to context, participatory research, and multiple methods. That sensitivity to context is essential should be obvious: it is difficult to imagine a successful evaluation concerning migrants or members of ethnic minority groups, whether of a programme or of a single intervention, which does not take into account the context within which the programme is embedded, factors such as community and organization which affect individual behaviour (cf. Israel *et al.*, 1995, p. 369), and the cultural factors discussed here.

As for participatory research, an approach which would seem particularly adapted to meeting many of the challenges posed by evaluation of HIV/AIDS prevention and care programmes and interventions for migrants and minority ethnic groups is that of action research (cf. Power *et al.*, 1991). An advantage of action research for evaluating AIDS and HIV projects is that the polarization between 'doing' and 'observing' becomes reduced. Action research is able to give both short-term feedback and long-term evaluation, and it feeds back appropriate research data to inform and define working practices and strategies (Armstrong and Hutton, 1992; Stimson and Power, 1992). Israel *et al.* discuss in detail the growth of interest in participatory action research (PAR) (Israel *et al.*, 1995, p. 379) as an innovative approach to intervention and evaluation. They argue that PAR is:

1 a participatory process in which participants are involved in all aspects of the action and research;
2 a cooperative and co-learning process in which participants and evaluators both contribute to and learn from each others expertise;
3 a reflective process that involves 'conscientization'; and
4 an empowering process.

It achieves a balance between research, evaluation and action goals and objectives. There are a number of examples in the literature of various forms of PAR as it concerns AIDS prevention or care and minority ethnic peoples (cf. Bletzer, 1993; Adrien and Leaune, 1994; Manson Singer *et al.*, 1994), and it was built in from the outset of the project at PIAA. One example would be the way the project has used focus groups for Irish people affected by HIV. Such groups have been established to evaluate research results, but the groups also provide participants with a forum to discuss issues affecting their quality of life, and a form of support and empowerment. Feedback from the focus groups has offered a wider understanding of research issues, and the groups themselves have allowed participants to develop skills which have enabled them to become more widely involved in public meetings, presentations and other forms of communication. Pure participatory action research is expensive, and perhaps primarily appropriate for demonstration projects, but it is perfectly possible to incorporate many of the principles into evaluation programmes.

Whatever the approach, such evaluations will most often require a great deal of flexibility, and of working back and forth between several methods. Participant observation, for example, has been a key element of evaluative research at PIAA, as discussed above. The researcher employed was of the same ethnic origins as the community served, and located within the organization, which assisted in the development of trust. The other author has used participant observation in the evaluation of an AIDS prevention programme for people seeking asylum, at a difficult moment in the programme when staff had become afraid of a more structured and traditional evaluation approach. Both authors have worked back and forth between in-depth interviews and questionnaires, writing questionnaires influenced by interview data or focus groups, exploring questionnaire results in interviews, each phase influenced by the preceding one.

A key concept is that of rolling assessment. In rolling assessment the circulation and processing of information is constant, with each stage — such as assessment of needs, participation, evaluation, and provision of knowledge — informing the development of the next. The positions of research and practical workers are complimentary to each other: research is assisted by the contacts, links and trust built up in a frontline service, and can act as a mirror to it, identifying and reflecting the issues which come up through service interventions, process evaluation, and interviewing. In the Swiss situation, for example, results of evaluation research are regularly used by field workers in their presentations on AIDS to community groups, and have also been used to produce materials, such as a comic book with a story about HIV. The PIAA focus groups just mentioned are another example of such rolling assessment.

Conclusion

At this point it is worthwhile recalling some basic principles, enunciated in practically any publication about evaluation, and pertinent to migrants and ethnic minorities as well: evaluation should be part of routine good practice, built in from the beginning of a programme. Programme goals need to be clearly and specifically defined, with clear indicators to help measure progress towards them. It is essential that evaluation and programme are interactive and reflexive, working in tandem, with evaluation giving ongoing, meaningful and constructive feedback.

From the point of view of evaluation of programmes in the field of HIV/ AIDS with migrants as with other population groups, evaluators need to be able to tolerate uncertainty (cf. Aggleton *et al.*, 1992b). Evaluations need to maintain maximum flexibility, using multimethodology (Power *et al.*, 1991, Chelimsky, 1994); qualitative and ethnographic data, surveys and monitoring. Focus groups should be used much more than they currently are (see Forrest *et al.*, 1993; Kitzinger, 1994, 1995). We need to concentrate both on processes and on outcomes — one without the other is incomplete — performing a 'rolling' evaluation of rapidly changing needs.

Whether the evaluation is internal or external, it should work in synergy with the programme being evaluated; evaluation should be oriented towards both action in the field and towards decision-making. Similarly, both researchers and those establishing programmes have to find the just course between prudent waiting for information and guidance, and simple learning from mistakes. In a situation in which outcome may be difficult, if not practically impossible, to predict and measure, and in a new field such as this one, process evaluation is especially important, describing the *why* and the *how* of what is going on, *what* was done, how it was perceived and received. For programmes for migrants and ethnic minorities it is particularly important to demonstrate that the programme is acceptable to the audience being approached. The mere gathering of numbers should be avoided: counting numbers of people who have attended training sessions is far too similar to searching for one's keys below the street lamp because that is where the light is. The easiest thing to do, it is unlikely to lead to much understanding. It is far more important to describe the interventions that lie behind the numbers, and formulate hypotheses as to the possible reasons behind any changes, or lack therof.

Some fifteen years into the epidemic, and seven years into programmes for migrants, far too much of the literature concerning AIDS and migrants and ethnic minorities is still 'grey literature', unpublished and thus of decidedly limited possible range of access (Haour-Knipe, 1994). Those doing such research need to publish more, to present their findings at conferences in order to raise awareness of issues and possibilities (Hart, 1992), to subject their work to peer review, and to disseminate knowledge of good and less good practices. An added, and non-negligible, benefit may be to help a community-based organization negotiate more equally with external authorities, giving the organization a voice through written work and papers delivered at meetings and conferences. At the same time, we need rigour: there is no excuse for sloppy methodology or mere propaganda to pass as evaluation, even if intentions are laudable. Excellent studies, of various or mixed methodologies (large-scale questionnaires, action research, ethnography), many of which involve target communities at all stages of the research, are the ones that should be supported. It is now time to take stock, to assess, to develop common approaches where possible, and hypotheses as to what works well and what may work less well. It is time to find a context for the comparison of experiences, materials (e.g. interview guides, or tested questionnaires in Spanish, or in Swahili, or in Serbo-Croatian), methods, and problems in the evaluation of programmes of AIDS prevention and care concerning migrants.

In a final set of conclusions we start with indicators, and end up with solidarity. For migrants as for other populations, core indicators as to programme effectiveness include:

- Behaviours: effective management of risk and adoption of appropriate prevention strategies. Management of risk involves taking into account situations, and may imply empowerment. Appropriate prevention strategies include appropriate use of condoms and of sterile injection equipment. They may also involve individually decided use of HIV testing, abstinence and faithfulness.
- HIV/AIDS knowledge: accurate knowledge of modes of transmission and methods of protection. Such knowledge is necessary but not sufficient. It is rare today to find individuals of practically any culture who are unaware of AIDS and of the principal modes of transmission, but an especially persistent residue of false knowledge is the

stubborn belief that one can judge whether another is infected by his or her appearance or social position. The underlying assumption is that HIV could only affect 'others' — certainly not 'somebody like me or my friends'.

- Attitudes: cutting through denial, awareness of HIV and AIDS as a problem that could touch one's own particular community.

Most important here is solidarity, or non-discrimination. Probably the best indicator of programme effectiveness is that a foreigner, a migrant, or a member of a minority ethnic group who is infected by HIV or who has AIDS, not only has access to, but also feels free to come forth for the care and support he or she needs. If media campaigns for general populations may be ineffective in precipitating individual behaviour change (Darrow and Valdiserri, 1992), they are essential for raising awareness and promoting solidarity. And the latter is essential to making things safe.

Notes

1 The studies discussed here were funded by the Swiss Federal Public Health Office. Most were performed in the context of the evaluation of the Swiss AIDS strategy, under mandates from the University Institute of Social and Preventive Medicine, Lausanne. Special thanks are due to Françoise Dubois-Arber for continuous support during many of the studies described here, as well as for helpful comments during the preparation of this paper.
2 The research programme at Positively Irish Action on AIDS is supported by the European Community, which we gratefully acknowledge. I should also like to acknowledge the generous support of all at PIAA in the development of the ideas presented in this chapter.
3 Most of these have been collected by Tovar and van Duifhuizen, and are available through the AIDS and Mobility Project (see Chapter 8).

References

ADRIEN, A. and LEAUNE, V. (1994) 'The challenge of HIV prevention among migrants in Canada: A public health intervention model', Abstract PC 0297, Tenth International Conference on AIDS, Yokohoma.

AGGLETON, P., MOODY, D. and YOUNG, A. (1992a) *Evaluating HIV/AIDS Health Promotion: A Resource for HIV/AIDS Health Promotion Workers in Statutory and Voluntary Organisations*, London: Health Education Authority.

AGGLETON, P., YOUNG, A., MOODY, D., KAPILA, M. and PYE, M. (1992b) *Does it Work?*, London: Health Education Authority.

ARMSTRONG, D. and HUTTON, J. (1992) 'A systemic model for evaluating local HIV/AIDS health promotion programmes', in AGGLETON, P., YOUNG, A., MOODY, D., KAPILA, M. and PYE, M. (Eds) *Does it Work?*, pp. 41–55, London: Health Education Authority.

BLETZER, K. (1993) 'Migrant HIV education in the wake of the AIDS crisis', *Practicing Anthropology*, **15**, 4, pp. 13–16.

CHELIMSKY, E. (1994) 'Where we stand today in the practice of evaluation: Some reflections', presentation at the first conference of the European Evaluation Society, The Hague, The Netherlands.

DARROW, W. and VALDISERRI, R. (1992) 'New directions for health promotion to prevent HIV infection and other STDs', in CURTIS, H. (Ed.) *Promoting Sexual Health: Proceedings of the Second International Workshop on Prevention of Sexual Transmission of HIV and other Sexually Transmitted Diseases*, London: British Medical Association Foundation for AIDS.

FARRELL, M. and O'BRIEN, O. (1995) 'The lure of the city: Migration and drug use', in DICKERSON, J. and STIMSON, G. (Eds) *Health in the Inner City: Drugs in the City*, pp. 21–9, London: Royal Society of Health.

FLEURY, F. and HAOUR-KNIPE, M. (1993) *Les Programmes de Prévention du Sida Auprès des Migrants en Suisse: Monitoring 1991–2*, Document 82.7, Lausanne: Institut universitaire de médecine sociale et préventive.

FLEURY, F., HAOUR-KNIPE, M. and OSPINA, S. (1991) *Evaluation de la Stratégie de Prévention du SIDA en Suisse. SIDA/Migration/Prévention. Dossier Portugais et Espagnol: 1989–90*, Document 52.7, Lausanne: Institut universitaire de médecine sociale et préventive.

FORREST, K., AUSTIN, D., VALDES, I., Fuentes., E. and WILSON, S. (1993) 'Exploring norms and beliefs related to AIDS prevention among California Hispanic men', *Family Planning Perspectives*, **25**, pp. 111–17.

FULLERTON, D., HOLLAND, J. and OAKLEY, A. (1995) 'Towards effective intervention: Evaluating HIV prevention and sexual health education interventions', in AGGLETON, P., DAVIES, P. and HART, G. (Eds) *AIDS: Safety, Sexuality and Risk*, pp. 90–108, London: Taylor & Francis.

HAOUR-KNIPE, M. (1994) 'Migrant populations: The development of something to evaluate', *Médecine Sociale et Préventive*, **37**, 1, pp. 79–94.

HAOUR-KNIPE, M. and FLEURY, F. (1996) *Evaluation du Programme de Prévention contre le Sida auprès des Populations étrangères en Suisse: Etude 1994–5*, Lausanne: Institut universitaire de médecine sociale et préventive.

HAOUR-KNIPE, M., OSPINA, S., FLEURY, F., CHAIGNAT, C-L., LUCKE, A. and LOUTAN, L. (1995) 'Evaluation of an HIV/AIDS prevention programme: Newly-arrived asylum seekers', *AIDS in Europe: The Behavioural Aspect, Vol. 4*, pp. 191–8, Berlin: Editions Sigma.

HAOUR-KNIPE, M., OSPINA, S., FLEURY, F. and ZIMMERMANN, E. (1992) 'HIV/AIDS: knowledge and migrant workers', in AGGLETON, P., HART, G. and DAVIES, P. (Eds) *AIDS: Rights, Risk and Reason*, pp. 85–101, London: Falmer Press.

HART, G. (1992) 'Evaluating a needle exchange scheme for injecting drug users in Central London: Defining success', in AGGLETON, P., YOUNG, A., MOODY, D., KAPILA, M. and PYE, M. (Eds) *Does it Work?*, pp. 103–13, London: Health Education Authority.

ISRAEL, B., CUMMINGS, K.M., DIGNAN, M. HEANEY, C., PERALES, D., SIMONS-MORTON, B. and ZIMMERMAN, M. (1995) 'Evaluation of health education programs: Current assessment and future directions', in *Health Education Quarterly*, **22**, 3, pp. 364–89.

KARMI, G. and HORTON, C. (1992) *Guidelines for the Implementation of Ethnic Monitoring in Health Service Provision*, London: NE and NW Thames Regional Health Authorities.

KITZINGER, J. (1994) 'Focus groups: Method or madness?', in BOULTON, M. (Ed.) *Challenge and Innovation: Methodological Advances in Social Research on HIV/AIDS*, pp. 159–75, London: Taylor & Francis.

KITZINGER, J. (1995) 'Introducing focus groups', *BMJ*, **311**, pp. 299–302.

MANSON SINGER, S. *et al.* (1994) 'Ethnocultural communities facing AIDS: Chinese and south Asian immigrants' risk behaviours in Vancouver', Abstract 191D, Tenth International Conference on AIDS, Yokohoma.

McEWAN, R. and BHOPAL, R. (1992) 'Context, theory and practice in evaluating preventive health education about HIV/AIDS', in AGGLETON, P., YOUNG, A., MOODY, D., KAPILA, M. and PYE, M. (Eds) *Does it Work?*, pp. 23–40, London: Health Education Authority.

O'BRIEN, O. (1993) *Assessing the Impact of HIV on the Irish Community in Britain*, London: Positively Irish Action on AIDS.

O'BRIEN, O. (1995a) 'The mobility project: Developing strategies for working with migrant populations in Europe', in FRIEDRICH, D. and HECKMAN, W. (Eds) *AIDS in Europe, the Behavioural Aspect, Vol. 1*, pp. 231–9.

O'BRIEN, O. (1995b) 'Irish migration and drug use', in O'CONNOR, J. and O'BRIEN, O. (Eds) *Drugs and Anthropology, Anthropology in Action Journal*, Summer 1995.

O'BRIEN, O. (1995c) 'Irish women and HIV in crossing the water: Irish women in Britain', *Womens Health Newsletter*, **25**, February.

ONG, B., HUMPHRIS, G., ANNETT, H. and RIFKIN, S. (1991) 'Rapid appraisal in an urban setting: An example from the developed world', *Social Science and Medicine*, **32**, 8, pp. 909–15.

POWER, R., DALE, A. and JONES, S. (1991) 'Towards a process evaluation model for community-based initiatives aimed at preventing the spread of HIV amongst injecting drug users', *AIDS Care*, **3**, 2, pp. 123–35.

RHODES, T.J. (1992) 'Community based HIV prevention', *The AIDS Letter*, 20 February/March.

RHODES, T.J., HOLLAND, J., HARTNOLL, R.L. and JOHNSON, A.M. (1991) *Hard to Reach or out of Reach?: An Evaluation of an Innovative Model of HIV Outreach Health Education*, London: The Tufnell Press.

RIORDAN, S. (1994) *Evaluating a Community Based Initiative: The Drugs and Irish Mobility Project*, London: Positively Irish Action on AIDS.

SHTARKSHALL, R.A. and DAVIDSON, Y. (1995) 'Testing a policy decision: What can happen when you screen for HIV', in FITZSIMONS, D., HARDY, V. and TOLLEY, K. (Eds) *The Economic and Social Impact of AIDS in Europe*, pp. 207–18, London: Cassell.

STIMSON, G. and POWER, R. (1992) 'Assessing AIDS prevention for injecting drug users: Some methodological considerations', *British Journal of Addiction*, **87**, pp. 455–65.

THOMAS, S. and MORGAN, C. (1991) 'Evaluation of community-based AIDS education and risk reduction projects in ethnic and racial minority communities', *Evaluation and Program Planning*, **14**, pp. 247–55.

WATTERS, J. and BIERNACKI, P. (1989) 'Targeted sampling: Options for the study of hidden populations', *Social Problems*, **36**, 4, pp. 416–30.

YOUNG, A., PYE, M. and AGGLETON, P. (1992) 'Challenges for the nineties: Priorities and needs in the evaluation of HIV/AIDS health promotion', in AGGLETON, P., YOUNG, A., Moody, D., KAPILA, M. and PYE, M. (Eds) *Does it Work?*, pp. 129–39, London: Health Education Authority.

Chapter 16

Conclusion: Shaping a Response

Mary Haour-Knipe and Richard Rector

A book, like a programme, is an organic thing, growing, sometimes in unexpected ways. It shifts as chapters come in: one never quite knows the shape of it until all the particular pieces are in hand. Even then, new understanding appears as chance brings one article, one point of view, in contrast with another. In this final brief chapter we identify some of the themes that have emerged throughout the chapters as the book was being edited, and some we hope to see evolve.

Some of the themes were inevitable, built into the very way the enterprise was constructed. Others have come as surprises. It is worth recalling that the book has been constructed as an academic-activist enterprise. Although we did at several points consider rearranging them, the chapters generally discuss over-riding issues in the first half, then turn to notes from the field in the second. Some readers may find certain chapters difficult reading, while others will find that other chapters are not properly documented. These very differences reflect the many facets of the field, and render all the more striking the themes that keep reappearing.

Although migrants' particular risk for HIV was a theme that was downplayed in the development of the book, the factors that may render migrants particularly *vulnerable* to HIV was a *leitmotif* that nevertheless appears in practically all the chapters.[1] All the authors writing here, in line with advances in thinking about AIDS prevention, specifically and vehemently exclude any notion of 'risk group' as one might attempt to apply it to migrants, but the notion of 'risk situation' is more extensively discussed, especially by Carballo and Siem, Sherr and Farsides, and Sabatier. They point out that many migrants may live in unfavourable social and economic conditions in host countries, exposed to the social inequalities now well-known to be related to HIV transmission.

That *stigma* emerged as a theme was no surprise. It had been the anticipated focus of two chapters (Sabatier, and O'Brien and Khan), and it appeared as a theme in many others. The idea that migrants, who are by definition 'other', are uniquely vulnerable to blame for bringing disease has been extensively discussed, and claims that AIDS is brought by foreigners is placed in the historical context of blaming migrating populations for other infectious diseases. Two other chapters take this up as a sub-theme. Fear of stigma, or the perception that migrants must be protected is the central argument of Jöhncke's chapter, and is also discussed by O'Brien and Khan. The result of such overprotection is often to do nothing. The latter authors take the argument further, arguing that the migrant, who by definition is not 'us', is often placed in the globalized category of 'Other', a bloc, easy to deal with since without individual differences, distinctions of social class, gender identification, food preferences or any other finer differentiations.[2] Such treatment helps keep ethnic minorities invisible, especially — and here we get to the heart of our problem — segments of minority communities who hide and are ashamed.

Nor was it a surprise that 'human rights', 'screening' and 'border control' emerged as central themes. Complicated situations encourage simplistic solutions, and at least fifty countries have tried to tackle the problem of HIV by trying to block it at the border, attempting to control disease by controlling the people who may have it. Matteelli and El-Hamad set the stage with an excellent discussion of general medical screening of arriving immigrants (more specifically of people seeking asylum), and van Duifhiuzen and Louhenapessy, especially, touch specifically on HIV screening, but it is Goodwin-Gill's solid chapter that explores the legal and human-rights' bases for HIV screening in their full complexity. The lesson from Goodwin-Gill's chapter is that we are going to have to come to terms with the fact that there are no simple answers. What we do find in this chapter, though, are arguments to help law makers resist public pressure to be seen as doing something effective by passing laws discriminating against vulnerable groups. We find, too, the basis for more nuanced and more just decisions.

Another theme across many, if not most, of the chapters in the book is that of *care issues* as they affect migrants. Belgium was the first European country to become aware of the need to undertake AIDS prevention among migrants, and the service described in Louhenapessy's article is now a leader in the field of care. HIV and AIDS care as it affects migrants is also discussed from the point of view of the service providers by Jöhncke and by Matteelli and El-Hamad, and from the point of view of those affected by O'Brien and Khan, and by Narimani, Tovar and Gallé. It is here that we begin to glimpse the full complexity of how HIV/AIDS affects migrants, as we cannot talk about combating powerlessness and loneliness by networking (Narimani, Tovar and Gallé) without also talking about legal rights and migration policy (see Carballo and Siem), or the host of ethical questions raised (see Sherr and Farsides).

'Culture', of course, has been a constant theme: cultural differences and working across them. We have seen that wanting to know ever more about 'culture' can become a reason to do nothing at all, as discussed by Jöhncke, but also that a programme that fails to take culture into account in talking of HIV and AIDS with migrants will inevitably itself fail. The secret, examples of which are provided by practically every chapter, is to *involve communities* themselves, a secret so obvious as to have become a truism. There remains the problem of just how to do so. Van Duifhuizen lists several of the rules, and gives an overview of how the task has been accomplished in several European countries, and Burgi and Fleury go beyond description to address policy. They write of diversity within migrant communities, but it is O'Brien and Khan and also Brussa who take the idea further. O'Brien and Khan, for instance, remind us that racism and denial are also to be found within minority ethnic communities: a well-intentioned community-needs assessment may find itself face-to-face with equally well-intentioned community leaders whose best interests and heartfelt convictions are to deny that HIV could possibly touch their people. Some 'community leaders', rather than being gatekeepers, in fact, could more accurately be described as roadblocks. The key, where HIV and AIDS are concerned, is most certainly to go to — and thus through — those affected, as shown in the several programmes that have now sprung from within migrant communities themselves (see Narimani, Tovar and Gallé on networking). At least two more complex themes then enter the equation, the link between prevention and care, and stigma: it has to be safe for those affected to come out of hiding. A way forward is shown in the Swiss programme for migrants (Burgi and Fleury), one of the basic pillars of which is to start prevention efforts by promoting solidarity among migrant community general populations.

Two new themes have arisen from the book: a public health rationale for dealing with the most vulnerable, and migrant resistance resources. It has long been clear that HIV follows the world's fault lines, that there is a risk to societies as long as we allow people to fall through the cracks of health and support systems. Two such fault lines in Europe today are migrant prostitution and clandestine immigration. Matteelli and El-Hamad, especially, in their chapter on the latter, make a strong argument for providing care to migrants regardless of their legal status. Even if some cannot relate to human rights, ethical, or other 'soft' arguments for providing care to people who legally have no right to such care, they show us there is a public health rationale for doing so. We are not far here from conceptualizing health: 'as a resource held in common, like the oceans, a resource that may be threatened worldwide and that requires collective action to protect' (Christakis, 1990, p. 343).

As for migrant resistance resources, it was Westin who set the tone by putting migration in its historical context, reminding us that throughout history, people have been seeking new places, and perhaps new challenges. Brussa touches on a related theme, showing how what could be considered a serious handicap, the extensive mobility of migrant sex workers, can in fact be turned into a tool for reaching larger numbers of individuals. But it is Sabatier's chapter that evolved in perhaps the most surprising way. Migrants are very often vulnerable. They are politically weak, and most often lack an effective voice to influence policy makers and service providers concerning the crucial issues affecting them. We often talk about finding ways to empower. Indeed Sabatier (1988) herself had been one of the first to write about the risk of stigma, showing how stigma might hinder the setting up of AIDS prevention programmes for migrants. What started out as a relatively minor theme in the first draft of this chapter, which revisits such issues, developed over successive versions into a significant leap forward, from 'you have to work through the community' to showing the too-often-hidden resources that can be found within communities.

The various chapters reveal many paradoxes and ambiguities, and some of the authors take contradictory positions. Narimani, Tovar and Gallé, when talking about networking, for example, find that because of its special importance HIV/AIDS requires specific concentrated efforts, whereas Burgi and Fleury, in discussing a country programme, go in the opposite direction, away from specific focus on HIV/AIDS and towards more general health promotion. The chapters present various facets related to migration, but some can well be applied to other arenas in HIV and AIDS. The constant sub-theme on human rights, for example, is applicable in a very wide range of settings indeed, and many of the ethical (Sherr and Farsides), methodological (Haour-Knipe and O'Brien), care (Louhenapessy), and networking (Narimani, Tovar and Gallé) issues, especially, are applicable to other populations and other issues.

As stated in the introduction, in order to avoid dispersion we decided at the outset to focus on Europe. This proved to be a wise decision: the issues are complex enough even when limited to one segment of the world, diverse, but homogenous in its relative wealth. It was wise in another way, moreover. There has been a constant struggle to maintain the focus: keeping attention on Europe has been extremely difficult, especially for those dealing with overriding issues. We presented the optimistic interpretation of this in the introduction: our desire to talk about AIDS in Africa, or in Asia, or in Latin America, most certainly reflects the extent to which AIDS is a global issue. The less optimistic interpretation, but perhaps equally as valid, lies in a tendency to focus on the problems elsewhere, to the detriment of those on our own doorstep. That said, our hope is that the fundamental issues addressed here will be applicable to migrants on other continents. Time will tell if what has been written here can be useful for other situations: for single male migrant workers in South Africa; for women in Abidjan whose only way of supporting themselves and their children is by selling sex; for young people of either sex moving to urban areas of Thailand, or of Haiti, in search of work; for Black or Hispanic drug users in Washington DC; for street children in Rio de Janeiro whose struggle to survive may include sex work and drug use.

The Way Forward

Some key issues could not be addressed in this book, simply because nobody was working on them. Others have been raised as it was being written. Still others are certainly yet to be defined. Although the World Health Organisation and the International Organisation for Migration have retained migrant health as an important area of concern for addressing current inequalities in health, much more remains to be done. We have too often failed to recognize migrant vulnerability to infections associated with HIV. The international response to the epidemic as far as migrants' communities are concerned has far too generally been limited to the sphere of testing, and usually in order to exclude. The construction of 'Fortress Europe', in addition, makes a particularly worrying context for discussing HIV and AIDS in relation to migrants. International response must include support for programmes and services specifically targeting migrant communities. Two of the major themes that have grown out of this volume can help define the way forward:

1   there is a public health rationale for providing AIDS care and prevention to vulnerable populations of migrants; and
2   resistance resources may spring from within migrant groups.

These both need to be emphasized, and elaborated upon.

On the European level, there is need to take stock, to put together what is already known. There is need for a forum, a place to share experiences, materials, information, and from which to encourage those who have not yet done so to write, publish, disseminate research on HIV and AIDS and migrants or ethnic minorities, and information about programmes. Further afield, there is need to put together information about the numerous programmes and individuals who are actively and effectively sharing information and materials between countries of origin and host countries, especially when the former are developing countries. Information to some extent does, and most certainly should, travel back and forth just as migrants do. It should do so in both directions, for example, as when Europeans explore the appropriateness of sharing prevention materials, and as when countries of origin are able to share models of caregiving.

Too little is as yet reliably known about migrant health in general. Risks, resources, and the health status of migrant populations, those newly arriving as well as those already residing, must be monitored in an effort to accurately document needs. As for HIV and AIDS, just as in the case of women, the possibility of specific clinical patterns associated with HIV among migrants needs to be studied. Further studies, qualitative and quantitative, from medicine and from social sciences, are necessary in the field of immigration to ensure that effective policies are developed to reduce vulnerability to HIV and inequalities in the delivery of health and social services.

The responses of health and social service structures to the needs of migrant communities urgently need to be improved. Appropriate medical, mental health and social services must be developed. Personnel across fields of migration, public health and human rights, those in universities, non-government organizations, associations of people living with HIV, and associations of migrant communities, must link forces to improve reception and assimilation of immigrants. The linkage between care and prevention as it concerns migrants, especially, needs to be further explored, developed and theorized.

Even when limited to Europe, one book has not been able to cover certain themes. The HIV- and AIDS-related needs of migrants in eastern and central Europe, especially, remain to be explored. Additionally, the particular problems of some subgroups of migrants remain to be addressed, such as those of asylum seekers and refugees. Also unaddressed were HIV and AIDS as they relate to migrants in prisons.

A theme most definitely related to migration, enormous enough to be the focus of a book of its own, is that of the risks linked to war. Rape as a military weapon, child militia, global strife and displaced persons in Rwanda, Burundi, Nigeria, the former Yugoslavia, the Commonwealth of Independent States, Afghanistan, Sri Lanka, to name only a few, and the destruction of vital infrastructures (including health, social services and education) can only add to vulnerability to HIV, and the overwhelming sense of powerlessness experienced by many displaced people.

An approach beginning to be explored in the migration literature is that of examining the contribution of migrants, asking what they may bring to countries, economically, socially and culturally, as productive members rather than as potential or actual burdens. This approach remains to be developed, for example, examining the actual and potential contributions of migrants affected by HIV.

There is an entire economic and ethical debate yet to be held around the question of a country limiting access to migrants whose health care is liable to be expensive, letting in only the fittest, or those who can work. The ethical issues surrounding migration and HIV/AIDS are particularly complex and difficult. These should be explored from within the formal framework of structured ethical argument, including an ethics of individual acts and rights, social ethics and an ethics of the common good. Finally, it must be stressed that migrants, too, are protected by international law. The imbrication, especially, of migration, border crossings, and restrictions thereupon raise critical issues which will need to be further addressed in the coming decade.

Conclusion

A common theme throughout this book on migration and HIV/AIDS is that both present major challenges for migrant health, public health, legal and human rights, ethics, social sciences and economics. The nature and the extent of the challenges posed, in addition, to governments and communities, is yet to be fully charted.

The changing face of Europe has brought us to a crossroads. One road leads us on the path we have so far been travelling, thinking of migration in terms of 'them' and 'us', seeing public health in terms of protection, and conceptualizing AIDS in terms of the infected and the non-infected. What this book has tried to do is to identify some of the foundations on which the bridges can be built. It is clear that the challenges posed will have significant implications for some aspects of national development. A successful response to these challenges will depend directly on the commitment, timeliness and effectiveness of the policies and programmes adopted. Our hope is that readers may seek to translate the understanding they may have gained here into interventions to meet these challenges.

Notes

1 As discussed in the introduction, we are using the term 'migrants' loosely, as a general term which should be read as also referring to 'foreigners', 'ethnic minorities', 'minority ethnic groups' and so on.
2 Such thinking is subtle and pervasive, and also appears in scientific discourse, seen, for example, in studies of migrant health which categorize subjects in a binary way being from a 'host country' versus simply 'migrant'. It includes facile generalizations about 'these cultures' or 'migrant communities', sometimes made even by people involved in programmes for such communities.

References

CHRISTAKIS, N.A. (1990) 'Responding to a pandemic', in GRAUBARD, S.R. (Ed.) *Living with AIDS*, Cambridge, MA: MIT Press.
SABATIER, R. (1988) *Blaming Others: Prejudice, Race and Worldwide AIDS*, London: Panos.

Notes on Contributors

Licia Brussa, a sociologist, is general co-ordinator of TAMPEP, the 'Transnational Project for AIDS/STD Prevention among Migrant Prostitutes in Europe'. Her research projects and doctoral degree have been in the fields of female migration and work. On the request of the Dutch government, she carried out a research project in 1991 on trafficking and forced prostitution in Europe, which resulted in an expert report for a seminar of the Council of Europe on this topic. She is currently linked to the Mr A. De Graaf Stichting, the Dutch national centre for research, documentation, public information, policy development and advice on prostitution and related issues.

Didier Burgi, delegate on migrants' issues at the Swiss Federal Office of Public Health in Bern, is in charge of health promotion and prevention programmes (AIDS and, since 1995, legal and illegal drugs) aimed at migrants and ethnic minorities in Switzerland. He has been implementing and co-ordinating the Swiss federal AIDS prevention programmes and activities aimed at nonnationals since 1990. A clinical psychologist with a postgraduate degree in health psychology, he worked in South East Asia for two years for an international humanitarian organization before entering the field of public health.

Manuel Carballo is an epidemiologist who established and headed the Social and Behavioural Research Unit of the WHO Global Programme on AIDS from 1987 until 1990. Between 1994 and 1995 he was the WHO Health Development Adviser, based in Sarajevo. He is now the co-ordinator of the International Centre for Migration and Health (ICMH), based in Geneva, Switzerland.

Issa El-Hamad is a Jordanian who migrated to Italy in order to obtain a medical degree. He has settled there with his family, obtaining postgraduate degrees in oncology and in infectious diseases. He has worked as a physician at the Clinic of Infectious and Tropical Diseases of the University of Brescia for the past five years, where he has promoted the establishment of an outpatient clinic for migrants. Acting as co-ordinator of the clinic, which serves undocumented and illegal immigrants, he is directly involved in delivery of both curative and preventive health care for local communities. He has undertaken and published studies evaluating tuberculosis prevention for migrant populations. An active member of the Italian Society for Migration, he participates in a national network of non-government organizations supporting health care programmes for migrants.

Calliope C.S. Farsides, a medical ethicist, recently took up a new post at the Centre of Medical Law and Ethics, King's College London. Prior to this she was Director of the Centre for Contemporary Ethical Studies at Keele University. She was a member of the Biomed I project, 'AIDS, Justice and European Social Policy', and has published a number of papers on topics raised in that group. Her main research interest is in the ethics of palliative care.

François Fleury, an ethnopsychotherapist, born in Switzerland in 1947, holds a postgraduate degree in AIDS prevention and counselling from the University of Grenoble. He has carried out several studies, beginning in 1986, evaluating AIDS prevention campaigns for migrant populations in Switzerland with the Institute of Social and Preventive Medicine in Lausanne, and has presented various papers on this theme at international conferences. A member of the WHO European committee on mental health and multicultural societies, he has published several papers on mental health and migration. He works as a counsellor and psychotherapist with migrants living in Switzerland, and is a co-founder of the Appartenances Association in Lausanne.

Felix Gallé was born in Offenburg, Germany, in 1963. He studied political science, history and Roman languages at the University of Heidelberg, with a focus on the politics of development and Third World issues. He tested HIV positive in 1987. Since 1992 he has worked in co-operation with the Deutsche AIDS-Hilfe e.V., first on documentation of self-help activities in Latin America, then as a member of the NGO Liaison Committee at the IX International Conference on AIDS in Berlin in 1993. For the past three years he has been working as a project co-ordinator with AKAM, AIDS-Koordinierungs- und Aniaufstelle für Migrantinnen, in Berlin.

Guy S. Goodwin Gill is Professor of Law, Carleton University, Ottawa, Canada, and Professor of Asylum Law, University of Amsterdam, The Netherlands. From 1976 to 1988 he served as a legal adviser in the Office of the United Nations High Commissioner for Refugees (UNHCR), and during the mid-1980s he participated in the development of UNHCR policy on HIV/AIDS with respect to refugees and asylum seekers. He has published widely on refugee and migration issues (the second edition of *The Refugee in International Law* was published earlier this year by Clarendon Press, Oxford), and on a broad range of contemporary issues, including *Child Soldiers* (authored jointly with Ilene Cohn; Clarendon Press, Oxford, 1994) and *Free and Fair*

Elections: International Law and Practice, Inter-Parliamentary Union, Geneva, 1994.

Mary Haour-Knipe, a medical sociologist, led a European Community working group (Assessing AIDS Prevention) surveying HIV/AIDS prevention activities for migrants and travellers in European countries. She has undertaken and published several studies evaluating AIDS prevention for migrant populations in Switzerland, and is currently completing a longitudinal study of migration and family functioning. Other main research and publication focuses are on migration and mental health, stress, and social equity and health.

Steffen Jöhncke is a Danish social anthropologist who combines academic and practical work. Since 1987 he has carried out a number of research projects and consultancies on HIV/AIDS in relation to male sex workers, gay men, ethnic minorities, and social work in general. He has taught anthropology courses at the University of Copenhagen, and is currently a research associate of HIV-Danmark, the national organization of people with HIV, and of the Copenhagen Social Services Department.

Shivananda Khan, is founder and Chief Executive of The Naz Project, an HIV/AIDS and sexual health agency for South Asian, Turkish, Arab and Irani communities. The Naz Project currently has two affiliate agencies, The Naz Project (London), providing direct services to these communities in London, and The Naz Foundation (India) Trust, developing services in a number of cities in India. The Project has hosted several consulation meetings and conferences, and produced a number of reports, and has actively participated in European networking for ethnic minorities around HIV/AIDS.

Maureen Louhenapessy, a trained social worker who has worked in psychiatry, has been involved in the Brussels AIDS programme for foreigners described in her chapter since it's beginning in 1986, and has co-ordinated the prevention programme since 1993. Her work has included development and running of multicultural projects, social work with persons living with HIV, training of non-professional field workers (street kids, African women) and of health and social work professionals (in cultural approaches to AIDS prevention) and research.

Alberto Matteelli is a medical doctor with a postgraduate degree in infectious diseases, experience in southern countries, and a special interest in tropical medicine, travel medicine, and international health. For the past five years he has been a physician at the Clinic of Infectious and Tropical Diseases of the University of Brescia. He collaborates in studies evaluating curative and preventive health care interventions, and is currently engaged in two longitudinal studies: one on tuberculosis prevention among migrants, and the other on STD/HIV education among immigrant commercial sex workers. He also serves as a European Community advisor on STD/HIV prevention and control programmes in several African countries.

Petra Narimani was born in Germany. She was responsible for international issues for Deutsche AIDS-Hilfe, the umbrella organization of German AIDS service organizations, from 1986 to 1995. Since May 1995 she has been co-ordinator of AIDS and migration activities for VIA e.V., a national network of migrants' projects.

Oonagh O'Brien, a social anthropologist, is the Information and Research Co-ordinator at Positively Irish Action on AIDS where she is co-ordinating the European Commission supported Participatory Action Research Programme. She has been actively involved in the development of the European Ethnic Minorities and Migrants Network and her research interests are in ethnicity and health and reproductive health.

Richard Rector, is policy co-ordinator for Migration, Health and AIDS. He has served as an advisor on health policy and planning in more than 50 developing and developed countries. He has more than ten years of experience in HIV/AIDS, working as a consultant for the WHO/GPA, Norwegian Red Cross, IFRC (the League), community based organizations and national governments. A social worker and health educator by training, his main interests include development, human rights, migration, social equity, health and policy development. He is also a person who has lived with AIDS for nearly 14 years.

Renèe Sabatier directs the Harare-based Southern African AIDS Training Programme, which provides partnership support for 150 AIDS organizations. A social scientist with training in community psychology and organizational behaviour, she has worked extensively in rape and trauma counselling, in capacity-building for women's shelters, and in community health and rights organizations and coalitions in several Asian and African countries. She has directed advocacy and lobbying for women's health campaigns in Europe and the United States. Author of numerous publications on AIDS and development, including *AIDS and the Third World* and *Blaming Others: Prejudice, Race and AIDS Worldwide*, she is currently involved in research and organizing on human rights and gender aspects of AIDS, reproductive health and sexual coercion.

Lorraine Sherr is a consultant clinical psychologist and a senior lecturer at the Royal Free Hospital School of Medicine. She is an editor of the international journal *AIDS Care*, and also edits *Psychology, Health and Medicine*. She has written numerous texts on HIV and AIDS, such as *HIV and AIDS in Mothers and Babies*, Blackwell Scientific Press; *Grief and AIDS*, John Wiley and

Sons; *AIDS in the Heterosexual Population*, Harwood Academic Press, and is involved in a wide range of national and international research work on HIV and AIDS, including European Studies on Discrimination and Legal Services, Ethics, Scenario Analysis and Ante-natal screening policies. She was a founding member and Chair of the British Psychological Society Special Group on AIDS and HIV, sits on the International Organizing Committee of the AIDS Impact meetings, and holds a Churchill Fellowship for research into AIDS and obstetrics in Africa.

Harald Siem is an epidemiologist who, until mid-1996, was Director of the Medical Services Division of the International Organization for Migration. He is the Chairman of the ICMH Executive Committee, and has written extensively on the relationship between migration and health, and health policy.

Jaime Tovar, born in 1963 in Bogotá, Colombia, is a chemical engineer with a degree from Universidad Nacional de Colombia, Bogotá. He tested HIV positive in 1986. Since 1992 he has been living in Germany. In 1993 he was in charge of co-ordinating the First European Information-Exchange Meeting of Migrants, Ethnic Minorities and AIDS, held in Blossin, Germany. Since 1994 he has been working as a co-ordinator of self-help activities in the recently created migrants and AIDS project: AKAM (AIDS-Koordinierungs- und Aniaufstelle für Migrantinnen) in Berlin.

Rinske van Duifhuizen has a masters degree in health education. She is currently Manager of the 'Migrants and Refugees' Team at The Netherlands Institute for Health Promotion and Disease Prevention. She is also co-ordinator of the European Project: AIDS & Mobility, and has been involved in AIDS programmes for migrants and ethnic minorities, since 1988. She has acted as a consultant to the World Health Organisation on HIV/AIDS education, communication and information issues.

Charles Westin, a social psychologist and professor of migration research, has been the Director of the Centre for Research in International Migration and Ethnic Relations at Stockholm University since 1993. His work, mainly published in Sweden, is about various aspects of migration and resettlement, integration policies, discrimination, majority and minority attitudes and the rehabilitation of victims of political violence, torture and war. He is currently working on a longitudinal follow-up study of the Ugandan Asians who settled in Sweden in 1972, and on an international comparative study of ethnocultural youth. He is the co-ordinator of the UNESCO sponsored project, The Management of Cultural Pluralism in Europe, as well as of the UNICA working group on Racism and Xenophobia.

Index

acculturation 36, 37, 44
African Foundation for AIDS
    Prevention and Counselling
    (AFAPAC) 216
Agence Gouvernemetale de Coopération
    au Développment (AGCD) 155
Aides Association 154
AIDS helplines/hotlines 123–4, 126,
    144, 148, 169
  for Spanish community in
    Switzerland 140
  for Turks and Moroccans in The
    Netherlands 124
AIDS prevention and care programmes
    10, 93, 96, 118, 127, 129,
    136–206, 223, 231, 234
  approaches to 123–6, 223
    cultural and linguistic 114–16, 155,
      158, 164
    ethnic mass media 123, 125, 126
    group education 123–5
    individual 123
  criteria for setting priorities 140
  guidelines for working with sex
    workers 202–3
  levels of interventions 140
  methods 11, 231
  pre-testing of educational materials
    128–9
  principles of 11, 87, 142
  recommendations for 11, 114–16,
    131–3
  strategies 11, 146
  in the workplace 143
AIDS Service Organizations (ASOs) 95,
    112, 121, 128, 130, 131, 207–8,
    231
  and racism 108

AKAM 12, 217–19
Appartenances Association (Lausanne)
    150
asylum seekers See refugees and asylum
    seekers
Austria 12, 194

barriers 36, 137, 157
  cultural 110, 118, 157, 172
  language 87, 110, 157
  legal and economic 35, 87, 157
  linguistic 35, 87
  religious 110, 157
  social 87, 118, 157
behaviour 72, 203, 234
  analysis of 114
  stages in changing 137
Belgium 26, 77, 154–65, 178, 182, 208,
    224, 240
border controls 32, 75, 240
Bulgaria 28
Burundi 155, 159, 244

care-givers 159
case histories and personal testimonies
  Chipo, a Zimbabwean migrant
    woman on prevention and care
    98–9
  Danish health professional recalls his
    contact with an African woman
    with HIV 167
  Imelda, Zambian mother of five 93
  Joyous, on new women migrants 92
  Martha, Tanzanian market women 93
  Mr A, HIV positive Zairian 160
  Mr B, on treatment and care 163
  Mr D, on treatment offered to
    people living with HIV 161

251